495

an outline of
Psychiatry

an outline of
Psychiatry

Clarence J. Rowe, M.D.
St. Paul, Minnesota

Clinical Professor of Psychiatry
College of Medical Sciences
University of Minnesota, Minneapolis

Lecturer, Department of Nursing
College of Saint Catherine,
Saint Paul, Minnesota

Psychiatric Consultant
Saint Paul Municipal Court
Saint Paul, Minnesota

Adjunct Faculty Member
Antioch College

In collaboration with Shirley H. Mink, Ph.D.
and Walter D. Mink, Ph.D.

sixth edition

WM. C. BROWN COMPANY PUBLISHERS
Dubuque, Iowa

TO THE McNULTY CLAN...

Especially

Patricia
Padraic
Rory
and Kelly Michael

They've kept the wind at their backs.

Mirior Invictus

Contents

. . .Hail, horors! hail,
Infernal World! and thou, profoundest Hell,
Receive thy new possessor—one who brings
A mind not to be changed by place or time.
The mind is its own place, and in itself
Can make a Heaven of Hell, a Hell of Heaven . . . .

Paradise Lost, Book I, lines 250-256
John Milton

Introduction to the Sixth Edition

The initial edition of this book twenty-one years ago grew out of the author's intent to present psychiatry in understandable terms to students of nursing, physical therapy, occupational therapy and other paramedical groups. The editions which followed also reflected his consulting experience to industry, courts, social agencies, and schools as well. Those editions seemed to meet the needs of medical students, social workers, psychologists, counselors, and psychiatric fellows as well.

The sources of the material contained in this Outline are multiple. No special claim to uniqueness is made. The contents represent the author's experiences at the University of Minnesota College of Medical Science, University of Minnesota Graduate School of Social Work, the College of Saint Catherine's Nursing Department, and the Saint John's University Institute of Mental Health Summer Workshops in pastoral care and psychotherapy.

Classification of Mental Disorders follows the *Diagnostic and Statistical Manual of Mental Disorders*, second edition, seventh printing, 1970, American Psychiatric Association (DSM-II). In each section, the older terms are listed as synonyms for each of the new definitions.

A Psychiatric Glossary (third edition), 1969, American Psychiatric Association, has been a helpful guide in formulating some of the definitions.

A special word of thanks is due the following: Drs. Thomas G. Bieter, Robert F. Fischer, Richard G. Lunzer, and M. Robert Wilson for having evaluated parts of the manuscript; and Drs. Shirley H. Mink and Walter D. Mink for their critical comments as well as their written contributions to the manuscript, including the sections on Behavior Concepts, Assessment of the Psychiatric Patient, and Behavioral Therapy.

Acknowledgment is also rendered to Mrs. Judith Schoeller and Mrs. Patricia McNulty Rowe for the preparation and editing of the entire manuscript.

The continuing acceptance of the Outline seems to suggest that there is an increasing need for an abbreviated introduction to the subject matter.

Clarence J. Rowe, M.D.

Man's mind a mirror is of heavenly
   sights,
A brief wherein all marvels summed
   lie.

Robert Southwell:
CONTENT AND RICH (1595)

Etiology of Mental Disorders

I. **Hypotheses:** Two major hypotheses have been advanced to account for mental illness. The *psychogenic* (of psychic origin as distinguished from somatic cause) hypothesis regards mental disorders as inefficient and unsuccessful compromises in response to conflicts resulting from the reality demands of the environment and the demands of the individual's internal desires. The *somatogenic* hypothesis regards mental illness as resulting from malfunction of the central nervous system. This malfunction may be genetically transmitted.

   A. The psychogenic explanation of mental illness is much more universally accepted for the group of reactions referred to as the neuroses (maladaptive emotional states resulting from unresolved, unconscious conflicts) than it is for many of the reactions in the group labeled psychoses (major mental disorders in which there is a departure from normal patterns of thinking, feeling, and acting; commonly characterized by loss of contact with reality, perceptual distortion, regressive behavior and attitudes, diminished controls of elementary impulses and desires, abnormal mental content including delusions, and hallucinations; may be of organic or emotional origin).

B. Thus, the causes of many, if not most, of mental illnesses are sought in disordered interpersonal and intrapersonal relationships.

C. In the group of psychotic disorders which are customarily regarded as psychogenic ("functional") in origin, there is less universal agreement about the exclusive primacy of psychological factors.

   Some investigators believe genetic determinants are operative in schizophrenia and manic-depressive illness and cite the findings of twin studies to support this position. More recently, neurophysiological, neurochemical, and neuropharmacological investigations have opened new vistas to our understanding of behavioral mechanisms (e.g., see sections on etiology for schizophrenia and manic-depressive illness).

D. Some psychoses, such as those accompanying cerebral arteriosclerosis, brain trauma, or certain toxic states, are thought to be explainable chiefly on an organic basis. However, it seems unlikely that anatomical or physiological cerebral changes by themselves can account for emotional disorders. Previous personality makeup, established adjustive patterns, and intrapsychic factors seem to play some role in determining the clinical picture (e.g., brain damage may lead to deterioration or depression or paranoid psychosis). Thus, mental disorder should be viewed as a disturbance of the whole person.

E. Psychogenic factors are regarded as of chief importance in mental illness (except organic brain syndromes). Included are the following:

   1. Antecedent factors: Forces operating during the early developmental years (including parental attitudes toward the individual as well as environmental and cultural forces).
   2. Concurrent factors: Precipitating or immediate causes which may trigger or initiate the onset of an acute mental reaction. (Such feelings are often hostile, aggressive, sexual, or dependency.)
   3. Intrapsychic factors: From within the personality; for example, hostile or aggressive impulses.
   4. Extrapsychic factors: From the environment; for example, parental influences or social forces.

Emotional conflict resulting from the interaction of all these factors seems to be of most important etiological concern.

II. Other factors may play contributing or predisposing roles. Included in these are:

A. Heredity
   1. Heredity is an important determinant of intelligence.
   2. The incidence of schizophrenia is much higher in the offspring of schizophrenic parents than in the general population.
   3. The incidence of manic-depressive illness is higher among the offspring of manic-depressive parents than in the general population.
   4. Many kinds of dementia (organic loss of intellectual function) are familial or hereditary (e.g., Huntington's Chorea—a degenerative disease of the basal ganglia and cerebral cortex; Friedrich's Ataxia; porphyria (an episodic metabolic disorder characterized by the excretion of porphyrins in the urine and accompanied by attacks of abdominal pain, peripheral neuropathy, and acute psychotic manifestations).
   5. It should be kept in mind that pathological emotional states may be transmitted by the parents to their offspring through the influence of the parents neurotic behavior rather than through the germ plasm (familial, rather than hereditary).

B. Age: For example, adolescence, the involutional period, and the senium (period of old age) are periods of special stress, not only because of somatic changes, but also because of psychological stress.

C. Gender
   1. Among adults, more women than men with emotional problems consult physicians. The reverse is true of children and adolescents.
   2. Affective reactions, including involutional disorders, are more common among women.
   3. Alcoholism is much more frequent among men.
   4. Suicide: more attempts are made by women in the United States, but more men are successful.

D. Marital status: Mental illness is less common among married people than it is among divorced and widowed persons.

E. Occupation
   1. Conflict about accepting the authority of supervision may be a precipitating factor.

  2. Competition for promotion itself may precipitate an emotional disorder.
  3. Overwork is usually a symptom of an emotional problem rather than a causal factor.
F. Physical illnesses
  1. Physical illness may pose certain reality problems for a person in terms of being able to make a living, personal discomfort, etc. It also may pose emotional problems arising from the person's psychological needs and even the reactivation of repressed, unconscious conflicts—especially in relationship to dependency.
  2. Certain illnesses which require mutilative surgery may pose disturbances of body image.
  3. Certain endocrinal disturbances, such as disorders of thyroid, may lead to associated personality disturbances (e.g., hyperthyroidism may lead to tension and anxiety; hypothyroidism may lead to the production of apathy and lethargy).
G. Physical handicaps: These may serve as a focus of inferiority feelings which may be handled by the individual through undesirable defenses. However, many people with physical handicaps do not show any significant emotional problems attributable to the handicap.
H. Exogenous factors
  1. Some drugs and chemicals, such as alcohol, sedatives, narcotics, and industrial toxins may lead to brain changes which produce a delirium or organic brain syndrome.
  2. Infections: Certain infectious diseases may lead to the production of delirious reactions. Syphilis may produce central nervous system changes with or without mental disease.
 I. Deprivations and deficiencies
  1. Starvation, for example, may lead to personality changes (meanness, suspiciousness, withdrawal).
  2. Sensory deprivation: For example, toxic deliria with hallucinations following cataract extraction when the eyes are covered.
  3. Sleep deprivation may lead to personality changes (inability to concentrate, restlessness, apathy, etc.).
III. **Etiology is complex:** Actually, the etiology of emotional illness can be regarded as a complex and complicated interaction of hereditary, environmental, psychological, and physical factors.
  A. Some of these factors are probably inborn, some develop so early that they become an integral part of "basic" personality structure, and others become operative later on.

B. This can be represented schematically as follows:

Inherited potential + early environmental influences $\longrightarrow$

Well-developed defenses + subsequent stress $\xrightarrow{\text{may}}$ lead to

Emotional Illness.

C. The foregoing scheme includes all the possible etiological factors but it will be noted that psychogenic ones are stressed.

D. It is oftentimes very difficult to separate constitution and environment, particularly in the first years of life.

REFERENCES:

Bosselman, Beulah. *Neurosis and Psychosis*. 3rd ed. Springfield, Illinois: Charles C. Thomas, 1969, chap. I.

Kolb, Lawrence C. *Modern Clinical Psychiatry*. 8th ed. Philadelphia: W. B. Saunders Company, 1973, chap. VII.

Dynamic Concepts

I. **Introductory comment:** The human organism undergoes a process of physical development from the moment of conception (fusion of sperm in ovum), until it reaches maturity. In part, this process is influenced by genetic determinants, but also is affected at any point in its course by forces which may impair its goal, produce malfunction or limit functioning of all or part of the organism. These forces largely derive from the experience of the organism in his environment.

Similarly, the same person undergoes a process of psychological development (maturation) which is also influenced by his hereditary background and various environmental influences. Included in the latter are his parental relationships, his peer relationships, his cultural and social experiences.

II. **Personality development**
   A. Personality
      1. Definition: This word has been defined in various ways. Simply stated, we can say that personality is the sum total of the individual's internal and external patterns of adjustment to life.
      2. It is in part determined by one's genetically transmitted organic endowment, and in part by one's life experiences.

3. As the individual develops, he will exhibit certain changes in his behavior (thus, a newborn reacts differently to a given environmental stimulus than an adolescent or an adult).

B. Stages of personality development
   1. Although development really is a continuum, it often is divided into stages (phases) for convenience of description and discussion.
   2. The stages
      a. Infancy (first year of life)
         (1) Even though physically separated from mother, the child is markedly dependent on her.
         (2) In our culture, the mother or mother-figure is of prime importance since it is she who has primary responsibility for the care and protection of the infant.
         (3) The relationships during this period are very important because they are probably the basis for all later relationships.
         (4) Period of elementary socialization.
      b. Early childhood (second through fourth years)
         (1) Period during which the child develops further his neuromuscular adaptation, including bowel and bladder training, locomotion, etc.
         (2) Period of domestic socialization. (Includes the Oedipus complex: Up through the fifth or sixth year, the youngster seems attracted to the parent of the opposite sex and feels rivalrous toward the parent of the same sex. To this family triangle Freud gave the term *Oedipus complex*. It is not found in all cultures, but the concept does seem to be of dynamic usefulness in our culture, and it becomes resolved through the process of identification.)
      c. Middle childhood (fifth through ninth years)
         (1) The *latency period*.
         (2) Period of communal socialization (turning away from restricted family constellation toward other outside relationships).
      d. Puberty and adolescence
         (1) May be recrudescence of dependent and rebellious feelings.
         (2) Striking bodily and physiological changes.

(3) Sexual differentiation (Note: sexual maturity in the biological sense is usually not coincident with social maturity).

e. Adulthood
(1) Social role of the individual becomes established.
(2) Achievement and maintenance of comparative stability.
(3) Equated with responsibility.
(4) Ability to accept the ordinary consequences of his behavior.

f. Senescence and senility
(1) Gradual waning of adaptive powers.
(2) If persons have been resilient rather than rigid throughout life, they are more apt to adjust successfully in their declining years.

III. Dynamic concepts

Most of our current conceptions of behavioral development and psychopathology originated with the work of Sigmund Freud and the subsequent contributions of other psychoanalytically oriented observers.

Psychoanalysis is a term which has two meanings: (1) a collection of data based on observations which has led to a theory of abnormal behavior, as well as a general theory of normal personality development, (2) the name of a psychotherapeutic technique.

A comprehensive résumé of psychoanalytic theory is beyond the scope of this Outline. However, a few of the basic psychoanalytic concepts which have been found useful in general psychiatry will be listed.

IV. Sigmund Freud (1856-1939)

A. Although degrees of consciousness were recognized before Freud (Leibnitz in 1714; Herbart in 1816; Fechner in 1860; Helmholtz in 1866; and Hartman in 1869), it is Freud's account of unconscious mental processes which has had a profound impact upon society and science.

B. Thinking: Freud viewed thinking as having primary and secondary processes.
1. Primary processes: The psychological expressions of the underlying basic drives. They are assumed to be largely unconscious, present at birth, and thus can be considered innate. They are the more primitive modes of thinking. They are manifest in dreams but also are present during

waking life. Thinking at this level follows the *pleasure principle*—the seeking of pleasure and the avoidance of pain.

2. Secondary processes: These are the reasonable and acceptable ways in which the underlying basic drives are controlled and permitted expression. They are characteristic modes of preconscious and conscious thinking and follow the *reality principle*.

C. There are certain significant desires and drives which are repressed. These constitute the dynamic unconscious, and they resist conscious expression because of their basic unacceptability. (See repression under "Adjustive Patterns.")

D. An individual resists attempts to make these forces conscious through the use of defenses (see chapter "Adjustive Patterns"). This constitutes what Freud called resistance.

E. Transference: The displacement of feelings for significant people in one's earlier life toward the physician or therapist.

F. To help explain all of these phenomena Freud postulated a mind composed of the conscious, the preconscious (foreconscious), and the unconscious.

1. The conscious is composed of ideas, feelings, drives, and urges of which the person is aware. It is the scene of purposeful behavior.

2. The preconscious, which is midway between the conscious and the unconscious, comprises feelings, ideas, drives, and urges which are out of the individual's continuous awareness but which are readily available to his recall. For example: one does not think about what foods he had for supper last night but could easily recall this if asked.

3. The unconscious is made up of drives, feelings, ideas, and urges which are out of the individual's awareness. He does not acknowledge or label them.

G. Psychoanatomically, Freud delineated personality into:

1. Id: The unconscious part of the personality which serves as the reservoir of primitive drives (instincts). This is found in *all* humans and in modified forms in all other animal life.

   a. Eros: The name he gave to the creative forces. The life instinct. (Eros was the Greek god of love and originally represented the primeval power that created order and cohesion out of chaos.)

   b. Thanatos: The name he gave to the aggressive, destructive, or death forces. (In Greek mythology, Thanatos was the personification of death and the twin brother of Hypnos, or sleep.)

    c. Freud felt that psychological growth depended on a proper balance between these two forces with somewhat of a preponderance of the creative ones.

    d. Libido: The emotional energy broadly derived from these underlying instincts (psychosexual energy) and presumably present at birth.

       (1) Ego libido (narcissistic libido): Libido concentrated on the self. Primary narcissism is the original state of the newborn. (Narcissus was a Greek youth who fell in love with his own reflection in the water.)

       (2) Object libido: Libido that is directed outward toward another person or thing.

    e. To the process by which the unconscious primitive drives were vested with psychic energy, he gave the name *cathexis*.

2. Ego: The part of the personality which meets and interacts with the outside world. The "integrator" of the personality.

    a. It represents those functions which deal with the external world, but yet satisfy the underlying needs of the id through coping and problem-solving mechanisms.

    b. It is partly conscious and partly unconscious.

    c. The adaptive functions of ego are the defenses against anxiety (see section on "Adjustive Patterns").

    d. The opposition of ego energy to id energy is called *counter-cathexis*.

3. Superego: The censoring force of the personality. It is composed of the morals, mores, values, and ethics of the individual and is largely derived from one's parents.

    a. It is partly conscious and partly unconscious. (The conscious part of superego is called *conscience*.)

    b. Most of us are conscious of our moral and ethical beliefs but remember only a portion of training and experience which contributed to the formation of those beliefs.

    c. If the ego contemplates violation of the superego's code, anxiety results; if the person acts on the contemplated violation despite the anxiety, guilt feelings ensue.

    d. The infant's superego is primitive and undeveloped. It begins to develop in the second year and takes definite form at the age of four or five.

    e. The punitive aspect of superego concerns itself with prohibitions, self-criticism and guilt feelings.

    f. The nonpunitive, positive aspect of superego is sometimes separately designated as *ego-ideal*.

    g. An overly strict superego usually leads to the development of a rigid, compulsive, unhappy person. A weak, defective superego permits a person to express hostile and antisocial strivings without anxiety or guilt.

H. Libido development (stages of psychosexual development): Freud placed major emphasis on the development of adult personality in infancy and early childhood.

    1. Oral Phase: The first twelve to eighteen months of life are characterized chiefly by preoccupation with the feeding experience. Pleasure is derived mainly through the mouth. The early part of the oral phase, or sucking stage, is passive. The later oral phase, or biting stage, is aggressive.

    2. Anal phase: From the eighteenth month until the end of the third year, the infant's attention is centered on bowel and excretory functions. This is the first time the infant must adjust his behavior to the demands of others, and the foundation for superego development is laid. Expulsive and retentive phases are described in the anal phase, just as passive and aggressive ones are in the oral phase.

    3. The oral and anal phases considered together are called the narcissistic or pregenital phase because the libido drives that develop within the individual are satisfied within his own body.

    4. Phallic stage: This period extends from the end of the third year to the seventh year. The child becomes aware of his or her genitalia. During this stage, for the first time, the child's libido is directed outward and requires others for its satisfaction.

        a. Castration anxiety: Anxiety stemming from the feared loss of male genitals. It includes the childhood fantasy that female genitals result from the loss of the penis.

        b. Oedipus complex: This is the attachment of the child for the parent of the opposite sex, accompanied by envious and aggressive feelings toward the parent of the same sex. This complex in the girl is sometimes called the Electra Complex. Resolution of this complex is usually accompanied by identification with the parent of the same sex.

    5. Latency period: This is the stage between the oedipal period and the adolescent years. In general, the emphasis during this period is on recognizing and coping with reality.

6. Genital phase: The final phase of psychosexual development.
   a. It begins with puberty, but it implies more than a physiological capacity for orgasms; such as the capacity for object love and mature heterosexuality.
   b. The early adolescent stage is narcissistic in that selfish interests predominate.
   c. Following this, there is a temporary homosexual phase in which adolescents prefer to meet in same-sex gatherings.
   d. As adolescence progresses, attraction to the opposite sex begins to assert itself more strongly.

V. Alfred Adler (1870-1937)

A. Founded the school of individual psychology.
B. He placed more emphasis on the ego than on sexuality. He regarded organ inferiority as the most important etiological factor and felt that personality was determined by the adaptive push for superiority, or the drive to power. In this quest for power, a particular *life-style* evolves.
C. He regarded personality as developing from an individual's attitudes toward himself, toward other people (especially his family), and toward society.
D. He coined the term *inferiority complex* to describe the conflict, partly conscious and partly unconscious, which impels the individual to make attempts to overcome the distress accompanying inferiority feelings. Thus, the person who has strong feelings of inferiority may behave in a superior way or develop some special skill to compensate for the supposed inadequacy.
E. *Masculine protest* was his term for the individual's (both male and female) attempt to escape from the feminine, submissive role. (In women: the "tomboy," the tyrannical mother or wife. In the male: the Don Juan syndrome.) It may be derived from the subject's own uncertainty of his role.

VI. Carl G. Jung (1871-1961)

A. Jung's modification of psychoanalysis was called analytic psychology.
B. He stressed life goals and the role of introversion and extroversion in personality development.
   1. Introversion: Inwardly directed libido, reflected in the tendency to be preoccupied with one's self.
   2. Extroversion: Outwardly directed libido (away from one's self).

C. Like Adler, he minimized the role of sexuality in personality dynamics.
D. He believed that the libido was broadly derived from all life energy (not just from sex).
E. In addition to the *personal* unconscious, he postulated a *collective* unconscious (racial unconscious), believing that there was an inheritance of primitive racial ideas and impulses. Among these were:
   1. Autochthonous ideas—ideas originating within the psyche without external stimuli.
   2. Primordial images—a phylogenetic memory heavily ladened with mythological reference.
F. He believed that the unconscious had an archaic or genetic, as well as an experiential, aspect (archaism—the survival of "the ancient character of psychic contents and functions").
G. He described the persona and anima.
   1. Persona: The social facade assumed by an individual (so named from the mask worn by actors in ancient Greek drama which characterized the mood portrayed).
   2. Anima: The true inner-self or soul.
      a. Animus: The masculine component of the female personality.
      b. Anima: The female component of the male personality.
H. He believed that psychiatric treatment should deal with current problems and plans for the future as well as attempts to uncover past causal experiences.

VII. Otto Rank (1884-1939)
A. Proferred the theory of birth trauma (the process of birth produces primal anxiety in response to feelings of helplessness). Separation from the mother is the original trauma. Subsequent separations of any type are also traumatic.
B. He emphasized the sudden, violent change from the security of intrauterine existence to the uncertainties of the outer world. Every pleasure ultimately seeks reestablishment of intrauterine primal pleasure.
C. As the child becomes conscious of himself as separate from his mother, he develops conflict. The desire for separation leads to guilt feelings, and relieving guilt feelings becomes the central focus of treatment.

VIII. Karen Horney (1885-1952)
A. She focused on the dynamics of interpersonal relationships as the chief source of psychopathology.

B. She did not accept the Freudian theory of libido and emphasis on infantile sexuality. She stressed the principle of basic anxiety: The child's apprehension and insecurity result from relationships with parents who are overindulgent, dominating, erratic, indifferent. As a consequence, the child is left without a feeling of belonging.

C. Hostility and conflict are considered to be of basic importance.

D. Thus, Horney stressed the significance of social and environmental factors in personality development.

IX. Harry Stack Sullivan (1892-1949)

A. He described an interpersonal theory of personality (interpersonal relationships provide the experiences which are crucial in personality formation, both normal and abnormal). He coined the term *acculturation*.

B. He believed that personality evolves from the action of personal and social forces in the individual from the time of birth onward.

C. He viewed the *power motive* as underlying all other impulses and operating from birth onward in an attempt to overcome an inner sense of helplessness.

D. He conceived of anxiety in the infant as stemming from a disturbance in the relationship between the child and the mothering one.

E. His views owe something to both psychoanalysis and psychobiology. (See Adolph Meyer.)

F. Treatment must include management of the patient in his milieu (environment).

G. Social psychiatry has developed from Sullivanian principles.

X. Erich Fromm (1900-)

A. He regards man as being in continuous conflict with his environment.

B. His theory underlines the fundamental basis of character as being found in specific kinds of person's *relatedness* to the world.

C. The cultural environment must be considered in the treatment approach.

XI. Erik Erikson (1902-)

A. He described the identity crisis and identity confusion.

B. His contributions are built upon basic Freudian tenets (in this regard he differs from Jung and Adler who rejected Freud's theories and substituted their own).

C. He postulated that (1) side by side with the stages of psychosexual development described by Freud were the psychosocial stages of ego development; and (2) personality development continued throughout one's entire life and each stage had a negative and a positive component.

D. He identified eight stages in the human life cycle.
1. Trust vs. mistrust (corresponds to the oral stage and usually extends through the first year of life).
2. Autonomy vs. doubt (this spans the second and third years of life or the anal stage).
3. Initiative vs. guilt (the genital stage, age four to five).
4. Industry vs. inferiority (age six to eleven).
5. Identity vs. role confusion (roughly ages twelve to eighteen).
6. Intimacy vs. isolation (young adulthood; roughly the period of courtship and early family extending from late adolescence until middle age).
7. Generativity vs. self-absorption (middle age).
8. Integrity vs. despair (the individual's major efforts are nearing completion and there is time for reflection and the enjoyment of any grandchildren).

XII. Contributions of Adolf Meyer (1866-1950)

A. American psychiatry has been greatly influenced by Meyerian thinking.

B. He founded psychobiology ("psychobiology studies not only the person as a whole, as a unit, but also the whole man"). His theory was characterized as distributive analysis and synthesis. The patient, under the guidance of the therapist, critically evaluates the situations with which he is confronted and his responses to them and through discussion and reasoning tries to formulate a way of dealing with his problems more constructively.

C. This is a comprehensive or pluralistic approach to the understanding of mental illness. Thus, he emphasized the need to consider all pertinent information about the individual's life as a biological, psychological, and social organism. This is sometimes called holism, or the holistic approach (the understanding of the individual personality is based on the interplay of his inherited structure, his uniqueness, and the cultural pattern in which he lives).

D. He had a common-sense approach, and although he emphasized the importance of considering the total individual from all points of view, he did not understand the significance of unconscious factors. (He undoubtedly understood what Freud meant by unconscious but chose not to emphasize it.)

E. He spoke of reactions rather than diseases.

XIII. Existentialism

A. This school of psychiatry is based on the philosophy of Sartre, Kierkegaard, and others.
B. This theoretical approach stresses the "here and now" rather than the past in the evaluation of personality disorder.
C. Actually, this theoretical approach has had little impact on present-day psychiatry.

REFERENCES

Blum, G. S. *Psychoanalytic Theories of Personality.* New York: McGraw-Hill Book Co., 1953.

Ewalt, Jack R., and Farnsworth, Dana L. *Textbook of Psychiatry.* New York: McGraw-Hill Book Co., 1963, chap. IV.

Freedman, A. M.; Kaplan, H. I.; and Sadock, Benjamin J. *Modern Synopsis of Comprehensive Textbook of Psychiatry.* Baltimore: Williams & Wilkins, 1972, chap. VI, VII, and VIII.

Kolb, L. C. *Modern Clinical Psychiatry.* 8th ed. Philadelphia: W. B. Saunders Company, 1973, chap. II and IV.

Millon, Theodore. *Theories of Psychopathology.* Philadelphia: W. B. Saunders Company, 1967, part II.

The ideas of goblins and sprights have really no
more to do with darkness than light; yet let but
a foolish maid inculcate these often on the mind
of a child, . . .possibly he shall never be able to
separate them again so long as he lives; but
darkness shall for ever afterward bring with it those
frightful ideas . . . .Many children imputing the pain
they endured at school to their books . . .so join those
ideas together that a book becomes their aversion . . .
and thus reading becomes a torment to them, which
otherwise possibly they might have made the greatest
pleasure of their lives.

John Locke

Behavioral Concepts
By: Shirley H. Mink, Ph.D. and Walter D. Mink, Ph.D.

I. **Introductory comment:** The experimental psychology of learning
has been the source of many useful concepts and techniques which
have contributed to the understanding and treatment of psychiatric disorders.

Learning approaches interpret psychiatric disorders as the outcome of experiences in which inappropriate or maladaptive learning, particularly emotional learning, has occurred. A major assumption of learning approaches is that the same principles of
learning which account for the development of behavior disorders
can be applied to the correction of disordered behavior.

In this section some fundamental concepts of learning will be
introduced. Examples of treatment procedures based on these
concepts will be included in a later section on treatment in
psychiatry.

II. **Ivan Pavlov (1849-1936)**
   A. Russian physiologist who discovered classical conditioning
      during his studies of digestion for which he won the Nobel
      Prize in 1903.
   B. He showed that a reflexive reaction can, under proper training
      conditions be established to a stimulus which does not nor-
      mally elicit the reaction.

17

C. His famous experiments demonstrated that the salivary reaction which occurs reflexively to food in the mouth could also be trained to occur to a neutral stimulus such as a bell or a light.
D. The training procedures involve the presentation of a neutral stimulus (e.g., bell) slightly before putting food in the mouth which elicits salivation; repeated pairings of the neutral stimulus with the presentation of food will result in the occurrence of salivation when the neutral stimulus is presented alone.
E. Using the standard terminology of classical conditioning a conditioned stimulus (CS) such as a bell when repeatedly presented slightly before an unconditioned stimulus (US) such as a piece of food which elicits an unconditioned response (UR). Salivation will result in a tendency for the CS to elicit the response which is then referred to as a conditioned response (CR).
F. Schematically:

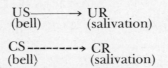

G. Some other classical conditioning phenomena.
   1. Extinction: Repeated presentation of the CS without occasional pairing with the US will cause a decrease in the CR.
   2. Generalization: When a CR is established to a CS there will also be a tendency for the CR to occur to a CS which is similar to the original CS.
   3. Discrimination: It is possible to train a CR to a CS while training the inhibition of a CR to a similar CS.
H. Classical conditioning may occur particularly in learned reactions which are mediated by the autonomic nervous system such as emotional reactions.
I. Pavlov noted a disorganization in the behavior of animals which are required to make extremely difficult conditioned discriminations; he called this phenomenon *Experimental Neurosis.*
J. Pavlov applied his analysis to the study of hysteria and obsessional neurosis and has been a major theoretical influence on contemporary Russian psychiatry.

III. John B. Watson (1878-1958)
A. American psychologist who formulated the methodological position in psychology which is known as *Behaviorism.*

B. He believed that psychology should be the study of observable behavior and should avoid references to unobservable mentalistic functions like consciousness.
C. Watson insisted that the experimental study of animal behavior could contribute to the understanding of human behavior and used Pavlov's principles of conditioning to explain human behavior.
D. He demonstrated in 1920 that fears could be learned by classical conditioning.
    1. A one-year-old boy named Albert became fearful of a white rat which did not frighten him previously when a loud noise was made behind him while playing with the rat.
    2. After a few trials Albert became fearful of any white rat without the noise and his fear *generalized* to other furry animals and objects.
    3. A few years later Mary Jones replicated Watson's findings and also demonstrated that a conditioned fear could be eliminated by conditioning procedures.

IV. B. F. Skinner (1904-   )

A. American psychologist who has refined Watson's methodological position and investigated the principles of operant conditioning; author of (among others) *Walden Two* and *Beyond Freedom and Dignity.*
B. He developed experimental procedures for demonstrating the way in which the consequences of an action influence the tendency to perform that action again.
C. His experiments have shown that occurrence in time *(contingency)* of a response followed by a reinforcing consequence such as food or escape from an annoying situation will increase the likelihood of the continued occurrence of the response.
D. The experimental training procedures involve providing an opportunity for an animal to emit an infrequent response such as pressing a lever—the occurrence of which results in the delivery of food (a reinforcer); repeated pairings of the response and reinforcement will result in an increase in the rate of response.
E. In the standard terminology of operant conditioning reinforcement may involve either the presentation of a desirable stimulus (positive reinforcement) or the termination of a noxious or aversive stimulus (negative reinforcement); in either case, the response which produces the condition is reinforced and will tend to be repeated.

F. Stimulus control of a response can be established by reinforcing the response only in the presence of a particular stimulus such as a light.

G. Schematically:

$$S\text{-----------}R \longrightarrow S$$

(light)   (lever press)   reinforcement (food)

H. Some other operant conditioning pheonomena.

1. Extinction: The repeated performance of a response in the absence of reinforcement will lead to a decrease in the occurrence of the response.

2. Punishment: The presentation of an aversive or noxious stimulus when a response is performed will suppress (but not extinguish) a response.

3. Discrimination: Reinforcement of a response in the presence of one stimulus but not in the presence of another stimulus will result in the stimulus in the reinforced condition becoming a *discriminative stimulus*; discriminative stimuli indicate that reinforcement will occur when responses are made in their presence.

4. Schedules of reinforcement: Varying the amount of time between reinforcements (interval schedules) or the number of responses between reinforcements (ratio schedules) will influence the rate and resistance to extinction of responses.

I. Operant conditioning principles have been used to analyze social learning, aggressive behavior, educational learning, and many other complex forms of behavior.

J. Many students and collaborators of Skinner have interpreted disordered behavior in operant terms and have developed training procedures for application in hospital and other institutional settings.

K. Recent studies have shown that operant conditioning may also affect autonomic responses as in the self-regulation (within limits) of heart rate and blood pressure.

V. **Some examples of a behavioral interpretation of psychiatric concepts.** (Many examples can be provided but these may be sufficient to illustrate the style of behavior analysis.)

A. Conflict

1. A behavioral interpretation of conflict stresses incompatible responses of equal or near equal response probability.

    2. The most compelling kind of conflict occurs when an approach response is elicited in the same situation where an avoidance response is elicited.

    3. An example of an approach-avoidance conflict might be experienced by a child who enjoys playing at a neighborhood playground but has been teased there by a bully.

B. Anxiety

    1. Anxiety might be interpreted as a autonomic nervous system reaction pattern which occurs in situations of fear or threat but becomes conditioned to irrelevant, coincidental or unlabeled aspects of the situation (as in Albert's fear of the white rat).

    2. Insofar as situations which signal anxiety are aversive, persons may be reinforced for learning ways to escape or avoid the situations.

C. Symptoms

    1. In a behavioral interpretation, symptoms are learned reactions which are the product of a history of reinforcement.

    2. If a symptom persists in a situation then something in the situation is reinforcing it.

    3. Symptoms can be altered by changing conditions of reinforcement just as with any other learned response.

REFERENCES

Hilgard, E. R., and Bower, G. H. *Theories of Learning.* 3rd ed. New York: Appleton-Century-Crofts, Inc., 1966.

Kimble, G. A. *Hilgard and Marquis' Conditioning and Learning.* 2nd. ed. New York: Appleton-Century-Crofts, Inc., 1961.

———. *Foundations of Conditioning and Learning.* New York: Meredith Publishing Company, 1967.

Symptom Formation in Mental Disorders

I. **Introductory comments**
   A. Symptoms in mental disorders represent expressions of the whole organism (not just the psyche or soma alone).
   B. The manifestations of mental disorder are the result of multiple forces, some of which are extrapsychic (from the environment) and some of which are intrapsychic (from within the personality).
   C. Thus, symptoms have cause and meaning.
      1. Symptoms represent the patient's effort to maintain his emotional equilibrium.
      2. In order to understand their meaning, one must know the patient's life history, including his needs and the forces (psychological, social, biological, etc.) which have been of importance in his own development.
   D. Symptoms in mental disorders are really psychobiological reactions.

II. **Somatic symptoms** (physical symptoms) in mental disorders are of two types.
   A. Physiological responses to conflict
      1. These are the types found in psychophysiologic disorders (formerly called psychosomatic disorders). They represent

physical symptoms that are caused in part by emotional factors and involve a single organ system, usually under autonomic nervous control. The physiological changes involved are those that normally accompany certain emotional states, but in these disorders the changes are more intense and sustained. Such physiological responses are also found in many of the anxiety neuroses (representing the physiological reflections of the anxious state).

    2. Such physiological responses are also found in many other mental disorders representing the physiological reflections of the particular emotional state such as anxiety, agitation, depression.

B. Symbolic expressions of underlying conflicts

    1. These are the types found in the hysterical neuroses (symbolic somatization) and are symbolic of the underlying conflicts.

    2. Examples are:

      a. Hysterical deafness as a defense against hearing something feared or forbidden.

      b. Hysterical paralysis as a defense against taking action.

C. Somatization reaction

    1. This is a term sometimes given to neurotic disorders manifested primarily as physical symptoms.

    2. Although it is usually synonymous with the term *psychophysiologic disorder*, it is sometimes considered to include the hysterical neuroses as well.

III. **Psychological symptoms:** These may be manifest in many ways.

A. Disturbances of affect

    1. Definition: Affect—mood or feeling tone.

    2. Anxiety: Uneasiness, apprehension, or fearfulness stemming from anticipated danger, the source of which is unidentifiable. It can be divided into degrees:

      a. Free-floating anxiety: Severe persistent, generalized, and unattached anxiety. Typically found in anxiety neurosis.

      b. Agitation: A state of restlessness and uneasiness; mental perturbation; typically found in involutional melancholia.

      c. Tension: Tautness, motor and emotional restlessness, and dread.

      d. Panic: An acute anxiety attack of overwhelming severity which leads to disorganization of ego functions (the word is derived from Pan the Greek god, who suddenly appeared to unsuspecting travelers in the woods, causing them to "panic").

3. Depression: A feeling of sadness, loneliness, dejection, or hopelessness. Typically found in depressive neurosis, involutional melancholia, and in the depressive type of manic-depressive illness. It must be differentiated from *grief* which is a state of sadness proportionate to a loss.

4. Euphoria: An exaggerated sense of well-being not consistent with the reality situation. Most commonly found in the hypomanic phase of manic-depressive illness and in certain organic disorders and drug-induced toxic states.
   a. Elation: Marked euphoria accompanied by increased motor activity.
   b. Exultation: Intense elation accompanied by grandiosity.
   c. Ecstasy: A feeling of intense rapture found in states of depersonalization and psychoses such as schizophrenia.

5. Apathy: Lack of feeling, emotion, interest, or concern. Impassiveness, unfeelingness.

6. Inappropriateness: Affect opposite to what would be expected. Observed in schizophrenia.

7. Ambivalence: The coexistence of two opposing feelings toward the same individual or object; they may be conscious, unconscious, or partly both. Found in many emotional disorders but especially in depressive neuroses and obsessive-compulsive neuroses.

8. Hostility (anger): Antagonism, opposition, or resistance in thought or behavior. Is closely allied to aggression. Found in antisocial personality and adolescent disorders.

9. Depersonalization: Feelings of unreality, strangeness, or altered identity. Found in schizophrenia, the depressive type of manic-depressive illness, and in certain neuroses.

B. Disturbances of memory
   1. Memory is composed of three processes:
      a. Registration: The ability to establish a record of an experience in the central nervous system.
      b. Retention: The persistence or permanence of a registered experience.
      c. Recall: The ability to recount a previously registered experience (from Freedman et al.).
   2. Amnesia: Pathological memory loss. This may be of organic etiology, such as is found in head injury; or, of psychogenic

origin, as seen in hysterical amnesia (see hysterical neurosis, dissociative type).

    a. Anterograde amnesia: Amnesia, forward in time.

    b. Retrograde amnesia: Amnesia, backward in time.

3. Fugue state: A personality dissociation characterized by memory loss and flight from the immediate environment. The individual escapes from his usual environment and during this state apparently acts purposefully. However, when he returns to consciousness, he cannot recall what he has done during the fugue. It is seen in the psychomotor equivalents of convulsive disorders and also in dissociative neuroses.

4. Hypermnesia: Abnormally vivid or complete memory, or the reawakening of impressions long seemingly forgotten. This is found in normal persons and in certain hypomanic and paranoid disorders.

5. *Déjà vu:* A subjective sensation that an experience which is really happening for the first time occurred on a previous occasion. Occurs in normal people, neuroses, psychoses, and organic brain syndromes.

6. Cryptomnesia: The appearance in consciousness of memory images which are not recognized as such but which appear as original experiences or creations (the reverse of *Déjà vu*).

7. Paramnesia: Distortion or falsification of memory in which the individual confuses reality and fantasy.

    a. Confabulation: A falsification of memory in which actual memory gaps are "filled in" by imaginary experiences (fabricated) which seem plausible and are recounted in detail. This is seen in organic brain syndromes, especially in Korsakoff's syndrome.

    b. Retrospective falsification: Unconscious distortion of past experiences to conform to present emotional needs.

C. Disturbances of consciousness

1. Definition: Consciousness is synonymous with awareness.

2. Confusion: Disorientation in respect to time, place, or person; accompanied by a state of perplexity. It is sometimes accompanied by disturbances of consciousness. It is commonly associated with organic brain syndrome and certain functional disorders.

3. Clouding of consciousness: A condition in which there is

impairment of retention, perception, and orientation. It is commonly associated with acute and chronic brain syndrome.

4. Dream state: A transient clouding of consciousness of intrapsychic origin in which the person is unaware of his surroundings and behaves violently or opposite to his usual pattern. It is seen in dissociative neurosis or convulsive disorders.

5. Delirium: A condition characterized by disorientation in all three spheres, obvious mood changes such as anxiousness, fearfulness or excitement, illusions, and vivid hallucinations. It may be caused by any agent or affection which produces cerebral metabolic insufficiency, which is temporary and reversible. For example, acute brain syndromes.

6. Coma (stupor): A state of unawareness and nonreactiveness. Profound unconsciousness. Found in certain organic brain syndromes and the stuporous form of catatonic schizophrenia.

7. Deterioration (dementia): Progressive loss of intellectual and emotional functions. This is found in degenerative diseases of the brain such as Alzheimer's disease; cerebral vascular disorders of the brain such as cerebral arteriosclerosis; and senile brain changes. Reversible deterioration is seen in schizophrenia.

D. Disturbances of orientation
   1. Definition: Orientation is awareness of one's relationship to time, place, and identity of person.
   2. Disorientation: Loss of awareness of one's position in relationship to time and one's surroundings or relationships with other persons. It is commonly seen in reversible forms in acute brain syndromes (toxic deliria) and in irreversible forms in chronic brain syndromes.
   3. Disorientation for time is the most common, followed by place and person.

E. Disturbances of perception
   1. Perception: The awareness and intended integration of sensory impressions of the environment and the interpretation of them in the light of experience.
   2. Illusions: Misinterpretation of real external sensory experiences (usually optical or auditory). These are frequently normal.

    a. Optical illusions: (e.g., heat rays shimmering on the road produce the illusions of pools of water [mirage]).

    b. Auditory illusions: (e.g., the roaring of the wind interpreted as the moaning of a human voice).

    c. Optical illusions are common in acute reversible brain syndrome.

3. Hallucinations: Sensory perceptions which have no actual stimuli.

    a. They are seen in people with toxic reactions from toxins, alcohol, drugs (including the hallucinogenic drugs such as LSD, peyote, or mescaline), as well as in people who have functional psychoses (as, for example, in schizophrenia).

    b. They may be auditory, visual, olfactory, gustatory, tactile (haptic), or kinesthetic (phantom limb is an example of kinesthetic hallucinations).

    c. Auditory hallucinations are common in schizophrenia.

    d. Colorful, vivid, visual hallucinations are found in acute brain syndromes.

4. Hypnagogic hallucinations (hypnagogic imagery): Mental images that sometimes occur just before sleep. Images seen in dreams which persist on awakening are called *hypnopompic*. These are normal and are found in healthy individuals.

    a. In *Oliver Twist*, Charles Dickens writes: "There is a drowsy state between sleeping and waking when you dream more in five minutes with your eyes half-open and yourself half-conscious of everything that is passing around you, than you would in five nights with your eyes fast closed, and your senses wrapped in perfect consciousness. At such times, a mortal knows just enough of what his mind is doing to form some glimmering conceptions of its mighty powers, its bounding from earth and spurning time and space, when freed from the restraint of its corporeal associate."

    b. Edgar Allan Poe was concerned with these sleepless dreams. In *Marginalia* he writes: "these 'fancies' have in them a pleasurable ecstacy as far beyond the most pleasurable of the world of wakefulness, or of dreams, as the Heaven of the Northman theology is beyond its Hell. I regard the visions, even as they arise, with an awe which in some measure moderates or tranquilizes the ecstasy . . . ."

c. Hypnogogic states are sometimes experienced by persons who are extremely fatigued but unable to find the time or place to sleep.

5. Eidetic imagery: The ability to produce vivid, accurate, and detailed visual after-images; "photographic memory." Such experiences are normal and are to be distinguished from hallucinations ("perhaps the artists have a greater eidetic power than most adults"—Franz Boaz).

6. Hysterical misperceptions
   a. There may be perceptual distortion in any of the sensory areas.
   b. There may be exaggeration of sensation or more commonly reduction of sensation. For example, in hysterical neurosis there may be hyperesthesia and hyperalgesia or conversely hypesthesia and hypalgesia.
   c. Macropsia: Visualization of objects as larger than they really are.
   d. Micropsia: Visualization of objects as smaller than they really are.

F. Disturbances of thinking
   1. Definition: Thinking—exercising the powers of judgement, conception, or inference as distinguished from simple sensory perception.
   2. Fantasy (phantasy): Fabricated series of mental pictures or sequence of events; daydreaming.
      a. May express unconscious conflict, gratify otherwise unobtainable wishes, or provide an escape from reality stresses.
      b. May serve as the basis for creative activities.
      c. A disproportionate preoccupation with fantasy may lead to harmful reality distortion.
   3. Phobias: Persistent, obsessive fears of specific objects or situations. Examples are: fear of height, closed spaces, dirt, or school. Typically found in phobic neurosis.
   4. Obsessions: Persistent, recurring ideas or impulses that remain in consciousness despite their irrationality. Typically found in obsessive-compulsive neurosis (also called ruminations).
   5. Preoccupation: Extreme or excessive concern with one's thoughts: engrossment.
   6. Delusions: Fixed false beliefs that are not in keeping with the individual's cultural or educational level. They may be:

    a. Persecutory: The belief that one is singled out for op-
pression, attack, or harassment.

    b. Grandiose: The exaggerated belief of one's own impor-
tance.

    c. Somatic: The delusional misinterpretation of physical
symptoms.

    d. Referential: The delusional belief that certain remarks
or behavior of others refers to one's self.

    e. Influential: The distorted belief that one can control
another person's behavior or thoughts. Most commonly
observed in paranoid and schizophrenic disorders.

       (1) Ideas of active influence: The psychotic person be-
lieves that he controls other people.

       (2) Ideas of passive influence: The psychotic patient
believes that he is being controlled by others.

    f. Nihilistic: The delusion of nonexistence of self, the envi-
ronment, or the world.

    g. Self-accusatory: Delusions of self-accusation.

    h. Other types of delusions including delusions of disease,
sin, guilt.

    i. Delusions are observed in various types of psychotic
reactions (both psychogenic psychoses and the psychoses associated with organic brain syndromes).

7. Blocking: Difficulty in recalling, or interruption of a stream
of speech or thought due to emotional forces which are
usually conscious. This is seen most prominently in
schizophrenic reactions.

8. Magical thinking: Belief that thinking becomes reality
("wishing will make it so") is a primitive prelogical thinking
seen in small children, dreams, and the thinking of
obsessive-compulsive neurotics.

9. Incoherence: Disorderly, illogical thought progression.
Sometimes manifested as garbled speech. Found in
schizophrenia, mania, and certain disorders associated
with organic brain syndromes.

10. Irrelevance: Thinking that is extraneous or inapplicable to
the subject at hand or the question asked.

11. Circumstantiality: A state of being incidental, adventitious,
and irrelevant in details. Found in those conditions where
the individual cannot distinguish essentials from nonessen-
tials. Commonly seen in mania or in some organic brain
syndromes.

12. Perseveration: A persistent, repetitive expression of a single idea in response to various questions. Found in some organic psychotic disorders and in certain types of catatonic disorders.
13. Stereotypy: The persistent repetition of a motor activity. Sometimes found in schizophrenia.
14. Psychomotor retardation: Slowing down of mental and physical activity. Most commonly observed in depressive states, but also found in some schizophrenic disorders.
15. Psychomotor excitement: Mental and physical hyperactivity in response to internal or external stimuli. This is seen in hypomanic and manic illness.
16. Flight of ideas: Skipping from one idea to another in quick succession, but without reaching the goal idea. Most commonly observed in the manic type of manic-depressive illness.
17. Autism (dereism): Persistent overindulgence in fantasy which ignores reality. Found in childhood schizophrenia.
18. Misidentification: Incorrect identification of other people. Found in certain psychotic reactions.
19. Intellectualization: The overuse of intellectual concepts and words to avoid affective experience or expression of feelings. It is found in the adolescent who wants to avoid underlying sexual impulses, borderline schizophrenia, and obsessive-compulsive neurosis.

G. Disturbances of speech and verbal behavior
   1. Blocking: See "Disturbances of Thinking."
   2. Flight of Ideas: See "Disturbances of Thinking."
   3. Logorrhea: Uncontrollable, rapid, excessive talking. Most commonly observed in manic-type of manic-depressive illness.
   4. Neologism: A coined word or condensation of several words to express a complex idea which has a special meaning to that person. Found in schizophrenia.
   5. Echolalia: The pathological repetition of phrases or words of another person. Observed in certain psychogenic psychotic reactions, certain organic brain syndromes, and in mental retardation.
   6. Echopraxia: The repetition or imitation of movements the subject is observing. Found in catatonic schizophrenia.
   7. Verbigeration: Meaningless repetition of incoherent words or sentences. Observed in certain psychogenic psychotic reactions and in certain organic brain syndromes.

8. Word-salad: A mixture of words and phrases which are incomprehensible and incoherent. This is seen in certain cases of schizophrenia.

H. Disturbances of motor behavior (disorders of conation)
1. Definition: Conation is the basic strivings of an individual as expressed in his actions and behavior.
2. Psychomotor retardation: See "Disturbances of Thinking."
3. Psychomotor excitement: See "Disturbances of Thinking."
4. Agitation: See "Disturbances of Affect."
5. Stereotypy: The persistent repetition of a motor activity. Sometimes found in schizophrenia.
6. Posturizing: The assumption of an unusual posture which is maintained over a prolonged period of time. Often the posture is an uncomfortable one. This is most commonly observed in catatonic schizophrenia.
7. Catalepsy: A generalized diminished responsiveness or immobility characterized by trancelike states. May be found in organic brain syndromes or psychogenic disorders.
8. Mannerisms: Stereotyped movements such as blinking, grimacing, gesturing. Found in schizophrenia and certain neuroses.
9. Negativism: Opposition, resistance, or refusal to accept reasonable suggestions or advice and a tendency to be oppositional. It may be passive or active. Its most extreme form is found in catatonic schizophrenia.
10. Mutism: A form of negativism characterized by refusal to speak for conscious or unconscious reasons. It is observed in catatonic schizophrenia, profound depressions, stupors of organic or psychogenic origin.
11. Automatism: Automatic, repetitious symbolic behavior, unconsciously directed. Observed in schizophrenia, convulsive disorders, and dissociative neuroses.
12. Compulsion: A recurrent compelling act which develops as an attempt to relieve obsessions or fears. Found in obsessive-compulsive neurosis.

REFERENCES

Freedman, A. M.; Kaplan, H. I.; and Sadock, Benjamin J. *Modern Synopsis of Comprehensive Textbook of Psychiatry.* Baltimore: Williams & Wilkins Company, 1972, chap. XI.

Kolb, L. C. *Modern Clinical Psychiatry.* 8th ed. Philadelphia: W. B. Saunders Company, 1973, chap. VI.

My apprehensions come in crowds;
I dread the rustling of the grass;
The very shadows of the clouds
Have power to shake me as they pass;
I question things and do not find
One that will answer to my mind;
And all the world appears unkind.

William Wordsworth: The Affliction of Margaret, Stanza X, 1804

Anxiety

I. **Definition:** A diffuse, unpleasant uneasiness, apprehension, or fearfulness stemming from anticipated danger, the source of which is unidentifiable.

II. **Features of anxiety**
   A. Anxiety is really an alerting process, warning the individual of impending danger and stimulating him to deal with the threat.
   B. It is a highly distressing psychic state, and for this reason one is usually unable to tolerate the symptoms for any sustained period of time. To deal with it, or manage it, an individual usually enlists one of the coping mechanisms or one of the defense mechanisms.
   C. Anxiety is similar to fear.
      1. Both are felt responses to danger and have similar physiologic reactions.
      2. However, anxiety, in the psychiatric sense, differs from fear in that the former is intrapsychic (from within the personality) in origin; is a response to an unknown or unrecognized threat; is conflictual; and is chronic.
      3. It should be noted that the distinction between anxiety and fear has been overdrawn and originally resulted fortuitously from an error in translating the word *angst* from

Freud's original work into English. Apparently Freud himself did not distinguish appreciably between the two.

D. Anxiety produces physiological changes in which the body is alerting itself and preparing for vigorous bodily activity (fight or flight).

1. Certain bodily processes are stimulated and others are inhibited. For example:

   a. The cardiovascular system is stimulated: The heart beats faster and blood pressure is maintained or elevated to force more blood to the muscles. The liver secretes sugar and the adrenals produce epinephrine.

   b. The gastrointestinal system is inhibited: Its secretions and peristaltic activity are reduced.

2. All of these bodily adjustments are a preparation of the organism for activity. Blood is temporarily removed from the gastrointestinal tract and made available to the muscular system.

III. **Role of anxiety in human adjustment**

A. Anxiety occupies a focal position in the dynamics of all human adjustment.

1. It serves as the driving force for most of our adjustments in life. For example, anxiety resulting from concern over security

   a. May drive one individual to accumulate excessive wealth.

   b. May stimulate another to plan a reasonable and realistic investment, insurance, and retirement program.

   c. May immobilize still a third individual to complete dependence.

2. The pattern for developing anxiety is inborn and always available. Evidence of this has been noted by child psychiatrists who have described the *universal* anxieties which are normally associated with the dependency relationship which the infant has with his mother (anaclitic):

   a. Separation anxiety

   b. Stranger anxiety

   c. Nocturnal anxiety

B. The coping mechanisms and defenses against anxiety are the basis of psychodynamics and psychopathology. These are discussed in the following chapter.

C. The consistent utilization of certain defenses leads to the development of personality characteristics or character traits.

IV. Components of anxiety: anxiety is present at three different levels.

A. Neuroendocrine: There is an increase in secretion of epinephrine.

B. The psychic manifestation is the sensation of apprehension and the cortical perception of discomfort (which includes both the appreciation of the physical responses as well as the apprehension).

1. Although the conscious aspect of personality perceives and realizes the apprehensiveness, the cause of anxiety usually escapes awareness.

2. Degrees of anxiousness

a. Free-floating anxiety: Severe, persistent, generalized, and unattached anxiety.

b. Agitation: A state of restlessness and uneasiness; mental perturbation.

c. Tension: Tautness, motor and emotional restlessness, and dread.

d. Panic: An acute anxiety attack of overwhelming severity which leads to disorganization of ego functions.

C. The somatic (motor visceral) manifestations are the resultant of the physiological responses of the various bodily systems to the increased secretion of epinephrine.

1. Dermatological response: The skin becomes pale, sweat is excreted, the skin hairs become erect, and there is a shivering effect of the superficial musculature.

2. Cardiovascular response: Usually tachycardia or palpitation; increase in systolic blood pressure; occasionally the cardiovascular response is one of decreased activity with resulting faintness.

3. Gastrointestinal response: The salivary glands are inhibited with resultant dryness of the mouth. In addition, the individual may show anorexia, nausea, vomiting, cramps, or diarrhea.

4. Respiratory response: May be rapid or embarrassed respirations. The hyperventilation syndrome may occur. (See section on psychophysiologic respiratory reactions.)

5. Genitourinary response: May be urgency or frequency of urination; dysmenorrhea, dyspareunia, frigidity, or impotence.

6. Vasomotor response: May be sweating or flushing.

7. Musculoskeletal response: May be manifested as trembling muscles (often first seen in the lips), dilation of the nostrils,

headache, backache, complaints of arthritis (or arthralgia), or various muscular or joint symptoms.
8. Pupillary response: pupils dilate (mydriasis).

V. **Pattern of anxiety responses:** There is great variance in the pattern of anxiety responses in individuals. For example:
A. Some may have primarily *visceral* reactions evident in any one of a number of systems; for example, the cardiovascular system; the gastrointestinal tract; the genitourinary system; the respiratory system.
B. Others may have symptoms primarily of *muscular tension*. These individuals have symptoms such as backache, joint symptoms, or headache (from muscle spasm).
C. Others might have combinations of visceral and muscular responses.
D. Why different organ systems are involved in different patients remains incompletely understood.

VI. **Stresses that lead to anxiety:**
A. These are often highly individual and depend upon:
1. A person's individual vulnerability.
2. The nature of the stress.
3. The individual's ego resources, including his coping capacity and defense mechanisms.
B. If his ego is functioning effectively, he will adapt satisfactorily.
C. Anxiety can occur either:
1. From conflict between the external world and the ego (extrapsychic), or
2. From conflict between the instinctual drives and the censoring forces (intrapsychic).

VII. **Anxiety: normal vs. abnormal**
A. Anxiety is essential to survival. It is emotional pain that serves as a warning or alerting process, similar to physical pain.
B. It is not always abnormal. Whether it is normal depends upon the causal circumstances, the intensity, and duration.
C. If it is severe enough, one is forced to do something about it (move about, take medication, have a drink, see a physician, etc.).
D. Anxiety is often a protective symptom. As a matter of fact, one could regard an emotional world without anxiety as being very similar to a physical world without friction.
E. During personality development various adjustive mechanisms evolve to protect the individual from anxiety.

F. As with physical pain, anxiety can be pathological and is so regarded:
   1. When it is triggered without a known cause or when it is precipitated by a minor event; or
   2. When it is unduly persistent and severe.
G. Cultural factors are influential in the production of anxiety (including religion, education, one's value system, and one's degree of sociocultural integration).

VIII. **Anxiety-reducing efforts**
   A. Because anxiety is a highly distressing state, an individual usually takes certain action in an effort to be rid of it or reduce it.
      1. Conscious attempts are often called coping mechanisms.
      2. Unconscious mechanisms are usually called the defenses against anxiety.
   B. Since most of the common clinical syndromes in psychiatry, with the exception of organic brain syndromes, are based on these mechanisms, they will be reviewed briefly in the following chapter before discussing the individual psychiatric disorders.

REFERENCES

Eaton, M. T., Jr., and Peterson, M. H. *Psychiatry.* 2nd ed. Flushing, New York: Medical Examination Publishing Company, 1969, pp. 15 and 16.

Freedman, A. M.; Kaplan, H. I.; and Sadock, Benjamin J. *Modern Synopsis of Comprehensive Textbook of Modern Psychiatry.* Baltimore: Williams & Wilkins Company, 1972, chap. 37.

Kolb, L. C. *Modern Clinical Psychiatry.* 8th ed. Philadelphia: W. B. Saunders Company, 1973, chap. V and VI.

Solomon, P., and Patch, V. D., eds. *Handbook of Psychiatry.* 2nd ed. Los Altos, California: Lang Medical Publications, 1971, chap. V.

Once more unto the breach, dear friends, once more;
Or close the wall up with our English dead!
In peace there's nothing so becomes a man
As modest stillness and humility:
But when the blast of war blows in our ears,
Then imitate the action of the tiger;
Stiffen the sinews, summon up the blood,
Disguise fair nature with hard-favour'd rage;
Then lend the eye a terrible aspect;
Let it pry through the portage of the head
Like the brass cannon; let the brow o'erwhelm it
As fearfully as doth a galled rock
O'erhang and jutty his confounded base,
Swill'd with the wild and wasteful ocean.
Now set the teeth and stretch the nostril wide,
Hold hard the breath, and bend up every spirit
To his full height! On, on, you noblest English!

Shakespeare: KING HENRY V

Adjustive Patterns
Coping Mechanisms—Defenses Against Anxiety

I. Introduction

A. An individual usually comports himself in a fairly predictable, consistent fashion. Although there may be some variation in his behavior, his psychological adaptation is generally in a state of equilibrium. Such a state of emotional poise usually results from his having accumulated a store of problem-solving mechanisms during the period of growth and development. Thus, when he is confronted with the usual life stresses, he has a variety of adjustive patterns which aid him in adapting to conflict and frustration in an effectual way.

B. Most of one's daily frustrations and conflicts can be resolved by conscious, deliberate coping mechanisms. Those more complex frustrations and conflicts are dealt with largely through unconscious defense mechanisms.

C. We all use defense mechanisms continuously. They are not of themselves pathological unless they are overused to a degree that they distort reality. As a matter of fact, oftentimes such defense mechanisms can result in gains for the person in his adjustment efforts; for example, constructive sublimation may result in highly successful vocational adjustment.

D. They are automatic—not planned; and are economical—not wasted.

   E. Defenses have a purpose: They keep us from being anxious.

   F. They are seen in normal and abnormal adjustments and can be regarded as protective devices.

   G. A learning interpretation of defense mechanisms would stress their effectiveness as avoidance or escape reactions which are reinforced by the reduction or termination of aversive stimulation, such as anxiety.

   H. Defenses are of two types:

     1. Successful: Those which abolish the need for immediate gratification or find substitute gratifications. Some authorities use the term *sublimation* to apply to successful defenses.

     2. Unsuccessful: Those defenses which do not do what is described in *1*, and hence do not resolve the conflict and the continuing need for the defense. (Thus, there is a repetition of the defense.)

   I. Synonyms for defenses against anxiety: Mental mechanisms, mental dynamisms, or ego defense mechanisms.

  II. Definition: Defense mechanisms are specific, unconscious, intrapsychic adjustive efforts which are utilized to resolve emotional conflict and free the individual from anxiety.

III. Defense mechanisms vs. conscious control: Defense mechanisms are out of awareness. We are unaware of them as long as they are working well. Conscious efforts are regarded as coping mechanisms.

IV. Specific defenses

   A. Repression: The involuntary, automatic banishment of unacceptable ideas or impulses into the unconscious (motivated unconscious forgetting).

     1. Psychogenetically this is the earliest type of defense available to the individual and is usually considered the principal defense in early years. It is the best known of all the ego defenses and one of the most commonly employed.

     2. It retains the position of a centrality that it was alloted by Freud in relation to ego defenses and symptom formation.

     3. It is sometimes used as a generic term for all defense mechanisms. It is a primary defense against anxiety and as such is considered the cornerstone of psychodynamics. It may be coupled with other defense mechanisms to permit the emergence of repressed material in disguised form.

    a. Repression plus displacement (focalization) to produce phobic responses.

    For example, the thirty-six-year-old mother who developed a phobia that her two-year-old daughter would contract a serious illness, as a defense against repressed hostility toward, and rejection of, the girl.

    b. Repression plus conversion (symbolic somatization) to produce a hysterical response.

    For example, the twenty-year-old soldier who developed a paralysis of his right hand when firing on the rifle range, as a defense against repressed hostility toward his father who had abandoned the family.

3. Conflicts that remain repressed are unchanged in quality and intensity. They constantly seek expression.
4. Not all repressed conflicts cause psychopathology in the individual. Repression is a frequently used defense mechanism in our lives. Only if symptoms of abnormal behavior result is it considered pathological.

B. Suppression: The voluntary, intentional relegation of unacceptable ideas or impulses to the foreconscious (preconscious). This is conscious forgetting.

1. Technically, since this is a conscious process, it is not considered a true defense mechanism by many authorities.
2. The conflict can be readily recalled since it does remain in the foreconscious.
3. This is a commonly employed coping mechanism of normal personalities.
4. Conscious control requires a strong ego.
5. Examples of suppression:

    a. The man who behaved foolishly under the influence of alcohol the previous evening may consciously try to forget about his behavior the following day.

    b. The student who wishes to study for an examination may consciously set aside distracting fantasies.

C. Regression: The return to an earlier level of emotional adjustment at which gratification was assured.

1. It may be partial, total, or symbolic.
2. All neurotic symptoms have a regressive aspect to a certain extent since mature modes of adjustment are replaced by behavior or symptomatology which represents a reversion to a lower level of adjustment.
3. Regression is not a desirable adaptation since in the process some developmental maturity is lost.

4. Examples of regression:
   a. Occurs normally in play and sleep.
   b. A toilet-trained, firstborn child may temporarily lose bladder and bowel control in response to the arrival of a second child in the family.
   c. A man promoted to a position of increased responsibility may have underlying uncertainty, insecurity, and indecision rearoused and reactivated, and hence ask to be returned to his old job.
   d. A person hospitalized for any kind of illness may have underlying, unmet dependency needs rearoused and reactivated, and hence react to these by making unnecessary requests and demands for attention and care.
   e. Excessive dependence on oral types of gratification can be a return to the breast. This is seen, for example, in alcoholism.
   f. Schizophrenia represents profound regression in the psychological sense. In the more severe forms, regression is seen in all aspects of the individual's personality.

D. Fixation: The arrest of maturation at an earlier psychosexual developmental level.
   1. Some believe that fixation occurs when there is excessive gratification at a particular level.
   2. Others say that fixation results from excessive frustration at the given level.
   3. Examples of fixation:
      a. An overly close attachment to another person, such as, a parent.
      b. Persistence of enuresis into adolescence.
      c. The continued attachment to a nursing bottle beyond the oral period.
      d. Infantile behavior is sometimes seen in psychosis which may be interpreted as fixation or regression.

E. Identification: The unconscious, wishful adoption (internalization) of the personality characteristics or identity of another individual, generally one possessing attributes which the subject envies or admires.
   1. Identification plays a decisive role in normal personality development, especially the development of the superego (including conscience).
      a. Normally, a boy identifies principally with his father and a girl with her mother.
      b. Children often emulate other important parent figures;

for example, teachers, scout leaders, athletes, television and movie personalities.
2. It is to be distinguished from *imitation* which is a conscious process.
3. A person may internalize certain undesirable personality traits of parent or authority figures. This is sometimes referred to as *hostile identification*.
4. *Identification with the aggressor:* The unconscious internalization of the characteristics of a frustrating or feared person.
5. A severe pathological kind of identification is seen in the psychotic person who believes he is God or some other important personage.
6. This mechanism is operating in cases of *folie à deux*. (See section on "Paranoid States".)

F. Incorporation: A primitive defense mechanism in which the psychic image of a person is wholly or partially assimilated into an individual's personality.
1. It is a special type of introjection.
2. It is the primary mechanism in identification.
3. It is assumed to begin during the oral phase of personality development and to be related to the nursing experience.
4. An example: The infantile fantasy that the mother's breast has been ingested and has become a part of one's self.

G. Introjection: The symbolic assimilation (taking into one's self) of a loved or hated person or external object.
1. This mechanism is the converse of projection.
2. It is sometimes regarded as a form of identification. It is also closely related to the mechanism of incorporation.
3. It plays a fundamental role in the early development of the ego (it antedates identification).
4. It tends to obliterate the distinction between the loved object and the person.
5. Instead of expressing anger or aggression against another individual, sometimes people turn these unacceptable tendencies against themselves as self-criticism, self-depreciation, and self-accusation.
6. In depressive reactions, the individual directs unacceptable aggressive and hostile impulses toward himself; that is, toward the introjected object or person within himself (for further details of this, see the section on "Affective Disorders").

H. Projection: The attributing to another person or object,

thoughts, feelings, motives or desires which are really one's own disavowed and unacceptable traits.

1. To some extent this mechanism, like rationalization, misinterprets reality, and hence is potentially dangerous.
2. It is associated with immaturity and vulnerability of the personality.
3. In a mild degree, it is seen in many normal day-to-day activities: for example, alibiing for failures of all types (economic, love, etc.); the "blind referee"; the unfair supervisor at work; the prejudiced teacher who "dislikes" the student and gives him a poor grade.
4. In the novel *Main Street*, by Sinclair Lewis, Carol Kennicott takes a walk in Gopher Prairie shortly after her arrival in that town. Looking up the street, she experienced, "...oozing out from every drab wall, she felt a forbidding spirit which she could never conquer."
5. Many of us are often critical of our own shortcomings in other people, and as a consequence, tend to hold others responsible for our own difficulties.
6. In a pathological sense, this is the mechanism operating in paranoid states of all types (paranoid personality, paranoia, other paranoid states, paranoid schizophrenia, involutional paranoid state). If the ego becomes disorganized, it leads to:
   a. Delusions, especially those of persecution.
   b. Hallucinations.
   c. Ideas of reference.

I. Rationalization: The ascribing of acceptable or worthwhile motives to thoughts, feelings, or behavior which really have other unrecognized motives. One does something and invents a reason for the action. It can also be thought of as unconscious, retrospective justification.

1. Rationalization, which is an unconscious mechanism, is not to be confused with pretending or lying, both of which are conscious processes (in both of these, the individual recognizes that the "reasons" given for his behavior are fictitious).
2. Much of our behavior has multiple determination; that is, several motives are involved. When we "explain" our behavior by the most acceptable of these motives, we are rationalizing.
3. It helps one preserve his self-respect and avoid accountability and guilt.

4. There is oftentimes a minor element of truth involved.
5. Examples of rationalization:
   a. Punishment, either individual or legal, may be a rationalization.
   b. Imbibing extra cocktails may be a rationalization.
   c. The teenage girl who is not invited to the dance, but really wants to go, may say that she prefers staying home anyway.
   d. The "sour grapes" response is allied to rationalization. (This is based on the Fable of the Fox who strove to obtain some tasty grapes but failed miserably and crawled away, muttering it was good he didn't get them because they were sour anyway.)
6. This is a commonly employed defense, but it is self-deceiving and hence is potentially dangerous.
7. It can also be positive in that it enhances self-esteem.

J. Intellectualization: The overuse of intellectual concepts and words to avoid affective experience or expressions of feelings.
   1. Is closely related to rationalization.
   2. Found in:
      a. The adolescent who wants to avoid underlying sexual impulses.
      b. Borderline schizophrenia.
      c. Obsessive-compulsive neurosis.

K. Compensation: A conscious or unconscious attempt to overcome real or fancied inferiorities.
   1. Status seems to be an important need in all of us, thus compensatory behavior is common in everyone.
   2. Compensation may be:
      a. Socially acceptable, such as the blind person who becomes proficient at music; the paraplegic who becomes successful in politics.
      b. Socially unacceptable, such as the physically handicapped person who becomes a bully or a boor; the physically small person who becomes aggressive and domineering ("the small man syndrome" or "the banty rooster syndrome").
      c. *Overcompensation* is an exaggerated attempt at overcoming inferiorities.
   3. Also compensation may be considered:
      a. Direct: An attempt to achieve in an area in which one has failed.

    b. Indirect: An attempt to achieve in a different field than the field in which one has failed.

L. Reaction formation: The direction of overt behavior or attitudes in precisely the opposite direction of the individual's underlying, unacceptable conscious or unconscious impulses.
1. It is closely related to repression.
2. Excessive politeness or courteousness may disguise underlying hostility and aggression.
3. Overt oversolicitousness and overprotectiveness on the part of a mother may hide her hostile and rejecting feelings.
4. Submissiveness, excessive amiability, or excessive concern may be reaction formations against underlying hostility, aggression, or death wishes.
5. Compulsive meticulousness may cover up strong soiling impulses.
6. Don Juan behavior may mask underlying feelings of doubtful masculine identification.

M. Sublimation: The diversion of unacceptable, instinctual drives into socially sanctioned channels.
1. This is socialization of emotion.
2. It is a term sometimes applied chiefly to successful defense mechanisms.
3. Thus, sports and games may sublimate hostile and aggressive impulses.
4. Various types of creative activity may represent sublimation of sexual drives.
5. Vocational choice for many people may represent in part a sublimation of some underlying unacceptable impulses.
6. Since sublimation offers some gratification of the underlying instinctual drive, it is usually considered a healthy defense. It is often regarded as the most desirable of the mental mechanisms.

N. Denial: The unconscious disavowal of thoughts, feelings, wishes, needs, or external reality factors which are consciously unacceptable. (One behaves as if the problem does not exist.)
1. Dynamically this is the simplest form of ego defense and is closely related to rationalization.
2. The person may replace the rejected reality with a more satisfying fantasy.
3. Examples of denial:
    a. The small child who disclaims pain when his finger has been smashed in the door.

      b. The deaf individual who refuses to admit his hearing loss.

      c. The alcoholic who refuses to admit that he cannot drink.

      d. The dissatisfied employee who believes that a change in jobs will solve all of his difficulties.

   4. Denial is to be distinguished from *lying* which is a conscious process.

O. Substitution: Unconscious replacement of a highly valued but unattainable or unacceptable emotional goal or object by one which is attainable or acceptable.

   1. To be satisfactory, the substitutive activity must have certain similarities to the original forbidden one.

   2. Murderous or intensely hostile impulses may be replaced by some impersonal destructive act, such as striking a punching bag or shooting a target rifle.

   3. It is comparable to displacement.

P. Restitution: A supplantation of a highly valued object that has been lost through rejection by or death or departure of another object.

   1. It is really a special form of substitution.

   2. Example: A second marriage of a widower.

Q. Displacement: The redirection of an emotion from the original object to a more acceptable substitute object.

   1. Seen normally where hostility is transferred from an employer to some member of the family or some other object; the displacement of various feelings onto political figures or certain minority groups.

   2. Feelings of hostility towards parents may be transferred to parent surrogates or other authority figures.

   3. Is seen in phobic reactions where there is transference of anxiety from an unconscious conflict to an external focus.

   4. Is frequently seen in obsessive-compulsive neurosis. For example, handwashing may result from the displacement of feelings concerning moral uncleanness to dirt, which must be continually cleansed away.

   5. Is found also in the transference-countertransference relationship in psychiatric treatment.

R. Isolation: The separation of an unacceptable impulse, act, or idea from its memory origin, thereby removing the emotional charge associated with the original memory.

   1. Setting apart an idea from its attached original feeling tone.

   2. Although the individual consciously retains, or can recall, the painful memory in a traumatic incident, he has detached it from the original feeling that accompanied it.

3. This mechanism is commonly seen in obsessive-compulsive neurosis. For example, an obsession in which a person feels he might hurt or kill someone but not have the accompanying hostile or aggressive feelings; it is the basis of many compulsive rituals. Characteristically, the obsessive-compulsive person remains emotionally aloof from loaded situations.

S. Undoing: A primitive defense mechanism in which some unacceptable past behavior is symbolically acted out in reverse, usually repetitiously (symbolic atonement).
   1. It is a nullification by counteraction.
   2. It is the treating of an experience as if it had never occurred.
   3. It is closely related to reaction formation (magical expiation).
   4. Examples:
      a. An executive who has recommended that an employee not be promoted later makes complimentary remarks to the person.
      b. In an obsessive-compulsive neurotic, hostility at the beginning of an interview may be undone by ingratiating behavior at the end of the interview; handwashing may represent expiation for various types of antisocial or asocial activities.

T. Dissociation: The unconscious detachment of certain behavior or personality activities from the normal or usual conscious behavior patterns of an individual, which then function alone (compartmentalization).
   1. Seen normally in the executive who keeps his industrial life from interferring with his family life.
   2. Found in sleepwalking (somnambulism), sleeptalking, and automatic behavior such as automatic handwriting.
   3. Found in dual personalities; for example, *Dr. Jekyll and Mr. Hyde* or *The Three Faces of Eve*. Generally, the primary character is proper and moral whereas the secondary personality is hedonistic and impulse-ridden.
   4. Found in the hysterical neurosis, dissociative type such as, amnesia, fugue, and twilight state.
   5. Also found in schizophrenia where there is splitting of affect from mental content.

U. Symbolization: The unconscious mechanism by which a neutral idea or object is used to represent another idea or object which has a forbidden aspect to it.

1. There is a displacement of emotion from the object to the symbol.
2. Symbolization is based on similarity and association. The symbols formed protect the individual from the anxiety attached to the original idea or object.
3. Symbolization is the language of the unconscious.
4. Dreams are the most common examples of symbolization.
   a. Elongated or projecting objects are often phallic symbols.
   b. Openings or shrubbery may represent female genitalia.
   c. A ship, an ocean, or mothering-figure may represent the mother.
5. Various affectations of speech, dress, or gait may be symbolizations.
6. Certain psychotic symptoms such as hallucinations, muteness, posturizing, and stereotopy may have symbolic meaning.

V. Idealization: The over-estimation of admired qualities of another person or desired object.
   1. Is seen in the young man who exaggerates the qualities of intelligence and attractiveness in his girl friend.
   2. Is seen in the precinct worker who overevaluates the assets and underestimates the limitations of his announced candidate.
W. Fantasy: Fabricated series of mental pictures or sequence of events; daydreaming.
   1. Daydreams can express unconscious conflict, gratify otherwise unattainable wishes, provide an escape from reality stresses.
   2. Fantasy may serve as the basis for creative activities.
   3. A disproportionate preoccupation with fantasy may lead to harmful reality distortion.

V. **Introjection,** projection, denial, fixation, and regression develop during the first year of life. Reaction formation, isolation, and undoing are said to be related to anal conflicts.

VI. **The foregoing** are not all of the defenses against anxiety that have been described by various authorities, but they do comprise the principal mechanisms seen in normal personality development, in day-to-day adjustments, as well as in the major psychiatric syndromes.

REFERENCES

Eaton, M. T., Jr., and Peterson, M. H. *Psychiatry.* 2nd ed. Flushing, New York: Medical Examination Publishing Company, Inc., 1969, chap. 1.

Freedman, Alfred M.; Kaplan, H. I.; and Sadock, Benjamin J. *Modern Synopsis of Comprehensive Textbook of Psychiatry.* Baltimore: Williams & Wilkins Company, 1972, pp. 111-112.

Freud, Anna. *The Ego and the Mechanisms of Defense.* New York: International University Press, Inc., 1953.

Kolb, L. C. *Modern Clinical Psychiatry.* 8th ed. Philadelphia: W. B. Saunders Company, 1973, chap. V.

Solomon, P., and Patch, V. D., eds. *Handbook of Psychiatry.* 2nd. ed. Los Altos, California: Lang Medical Publications, 1971, chap. 31.

But Sun it is not, when you say it is not;
And the moon changes even as your mind.
What you will have it nam'd even that it is;
and so it shall be so for Katherine.

Shakespeare, The Taming of the Shrew

Classification
of Mental Disorders

I. **Introductory comment:** In general, the nomenclature in this Outline is patterned after the classification in the *Diagnostic and Statistical Manual of Mental Disorders,* second edition, seventh printing,
1974 (DSM-II). This manual, published by the American Psychiatric Association, reflects updating and revisions resulting from the
publication of the *International Classification of Diseases* approved by
the World Health Organization (ICS-8).

II. **Classification (specific psychiatric syndromes)**
  A. Neuroses (300): Includes disturbances in which felt or expres-
     sed anxiety is a major characteristic or in which the individual
     automatically or unconsciously attempts to control the anxiety
     by the use of various ego-defense mechanisms. Generally,
     these mechanisms produce subjectively distressing symptoms
     from which the patient seeks relief. Reality is not grossly dis-
     torted and personality is not grossly disorganized.
     1. Anxiety neurosis
     2. Phobic neurosis
     3. Hysterical neurosis
        a. Hysterical neurosis, conversion type
        b. Hysterical neurosis, dissociative type
     4. Depressive neurosis

49

5. Obsessive-compulsive neurosis
6. Neurasthenic neurosis (neurasthenia)
7. Depersonalization neurosis (depersonalization syndrome)
8. Hypochondriacal neurosis
9. Other neurosis

B. Psychophysiologic disorders (305): Characterized by physical symptoms that represent physiological expressions which usually accompany certain emotional states. However, in these disorders, the changes are more intense and sustained. Usually, a single organ system under autonomic nervous control is affected.

These disorders can be manifested in the various bodily systems such as: skin; musculoskeletal system; respiratory system; cardiovascular system; hemic and lymphatic systems; gastrointestinal system; genitourinary system; endocrine system; and organs of special sense.

C. Personality disorders and certain other nonpsychotic mental disorders (301-304): These are disorders in which the personality structure (character) is defective and in which deeply ingrained maladaptive patterns are evident. Such disorders are usually manifested by lifelong patterns of behavior and often recognizable at adolescence or earlier.

1. Personality disorders (301):
   a. Paranoid personality
   b. Cyclothymic personality (affective personality)
   c. Schizoid personality
   d. Explosive personality (epileptoid personality disorder)
   e. Obsessive-compulsive personality (anankastic personality)
   f. Hysterical personality (histrionic personality disorder)
   g. Asthenic personality
   h. Antisocial personality
   i. Passive-aggressive personality
   j. Inadequate personality
   k. Other personality disorders of specified types
2. Sexual deviations (302): This category is for individuals whose sexual interests are directed primarily toward objects other than humans of the opposite sex, toward sexual acts not usually associated with coitus, or toward coitus performed under bizarre circumstances.

1. Numbers in parentheses indicate sections of the DSM-II for reference.

        a. Homosexuality[2]
        b. Fetishism
        c. Pedophilia
        d. Trasvestitism
        e. Exhibitionism
        f. Voyeurism
        g. Sadism
        h. Masochism
        i. Other sexual deviations

3. Alcoholism (303): Characterized by alcoholic intake great enough to damage physical health, personal or social functioning, or when it has become a prerequisite to normal functioning.
        a. Episodic excessive drinking
        b. Habitual excessive drinking
        c. Alcohol addiction
        d. Other

4. Drug dependence (304): A category for patients who are addicted to, or who are dependent on, drugs other than alcohol, tobacco, and ordinary caffeine-containing beverages. It includes dependence on opium alkaloids and their derivatives; synthetic analgesics; barbiturates; hypnotics, sedatives, or tranquilizers; cocaine, marijuana; psychostimulants; hallucinogens (such as LSD).

D. Transient situational disturbances (307): These disorders are more or less transient in character and appear to represent an acute reaction to an overwhelming environmental stress in an individual without evident underlying mental disorders. The symptoms subside when the stress diminishes. Disorders in this category are classified according to the patient's developmental stage as follows:

1. Adjustment reaction of infancy
2. Adjustment reaction of childhood
3. Adjustment reaction of adolescence
4. Adjustment reaction of adult life
5. Adjustment reaction of late life

---

2. In December, 1973 the Board of Trustees of the American Psychiatric Association substituted for homosexuality a new definition and category: *Sexual Orientation Disturbance.* This category is for individuals whose sexual interests are directed primarily toward people of the same sex and who are either disturbed by, in conflict with, or wish to change their sexual orientation. This diagnostic category is distinguished from homosexuality, which by itself, does not necessarily constitute a psychiatric disorder. This decision was upheld by a substantial majority in a referendum of the voting members of the association in May, 1974.

E. Special symptoms (306): This category is for the occasional patient whose psychopathology is manifested by a single specific symptom.
1. Speech disturbance
2. Specific learning disturbance
3. Tic
4. Other psychomotor disorder
5. Disorder of sleep
6. Feeding disturbance
7. Enuresis
8. Encopresis
9. Cephalalgia
10. Other special symptoms
F. Behavior disorders of childhood and adolescence (308): This category is reserved for disorders occurring in childhood and adolescence that are more stable, internalized, and resistant to treatment than transient situational disturbances, but less so than psychoses, neuroses, and personality disorders.
1. Hyperkenetic reaction of childhood (or adolescence)
2. Withdrawing reaction of childhood (or adolescence)
3. Overanxious reaction of childhood (or adolescence)
4. Run-away reaction of childhood (or adolescence)
5. Unsocialized aggressive reaction of childhood (or adolescence)
6. Group delinquent reaction of childhood (or adolescence)
7. Other reaction of childhood (or adolescence)
G. Conditions without manifest psychiatric disorder and non-specific conditions (316-318):
1. Social maladjustments without manifest psychiatric disorder: a category for individuals who are psychiatrically normal, but nevertheless have severe enough problems to warrant examination by a psychiatrist. Such conditions may either become or precipitate a diagnosable mental disorder.
a. Marital maladjustment
b. Social maladjustment
c. Occupational maladjustment
d. Dyssocial behavior
e. Other social maladjustments
2. Nonspecific conditions: a category for conditions that cannot be classified under any of the other previous categories.
3. No mental disorder

H. Psychoses not attributable to physical conditions (295-298):
   1. Schizophrenia (295): A group of disorders characterized by disturbances in thinking, mood, and behavior.
      a. Schizophrenia, simple type
      b. Schizophrenia, hebephrenic type
      c. Schizophrenia, catatonic type:
         (1) Excited
         (2) Withdrawn
      d. Schizophrenia, paranoid type
      e. Acute schizophrenic episode
      f. Schizophrenia, latent type
      g. Schizophrenia, residual type
      h. Schizophrenia, schizo-affective type
         (1) Schizophrenia, schizo-affective type, excited
         (2) Schizophrenia, schizo-affective type, depressed
      i. Schizophrenia, childhood type
      j. Schizophrenia, chronic undifferentiated type
      k. Schizophrenia, other
   2. Major affective disorders (affective psychoses) (296): Characterized by a single disorder of mood, either extreme depression or elation.
      a. Involutional melancholia
      b. Manic-depressive illness (manic-depressive psychosis)
         (1) Manic-depressive illness, manic type (manic-depressive psychosis, manic type)
         (2) Manic-depressive illness, depressed type (manic-depressive psychosis, depressed type)
         (3) Manic-depressive illness, circular type (manic-depressive psychosis, circular type)
            (a) Manic-depressive illness, circular type, manic
            (b) Manic-depressive illness, circular type, depressed
      c. Other major affective disorders
   3. Paranoid states (297): Characterized by the presence of persecutory or expansive delusions without hallucinations and without schizophrenic behavior.
      a. Paranoia
      b. Involutional paranoid state (involutional paraphrenia)
      c. Other paranoid states
   4. Psychotic depressive reaction (298.0): A psychosis distinguished by a depressive mood attributable to some experience and without a history of repeated depressions or cyclothymic mood swings.

I. Organic brain syndromes: Mental conditions resulting from diffuse impairment of brain tissue function from whatever cause. These disorders are manifested by the following impairment syndrome:
   a. Impairment of orientation
   b. Impairment of memory
   c. Impairment of intellectual functions such as comprehension, calculation, knowledge, learning
   d. Impairment of judgment
   e. Lability and shallowness of affect
1. Psychoses associated with organic brain syndromes (290-294)
   a. Senile and Presenile dementia (290)
      (1) Senile dementia
      (2) Presenile dementia
   b. Alcoholic Psychosis (291)
      (1) Delirium tremens
      (2) Korsakov's psychosis
      (3) Other alcoholic hallucinosis
      (4) Alcoholic paranoid state
      (5) Acute alcoholic intoxication
      (6) Alcoholic deterioration
      (7) Pathological intoxication
      (8) Other (and unspecified) alcoholic psychosis
   c. Psychosis associated with intracranial infection (292): Included here are the psychoses associated with general paralysis, central nervous system syphilis, epidemic encephalitis, and other unspecified encephalitides and intracranial infections.
   d. Psychosis associated with other cerebral condition (293): Included are the psychoses associated with cerebral arteriosclerosis, other cerebrovascular disturbance, epilepsy, intracranial neoplasms, degenerative disease of the nervous system, brain trauma, and with other (and unspecified) cerebral conditions.
   e. Psychosis associated with other physical condition (294): Included here would be psychoses associated with endocrine disorders, metabolic or nutritional disorders, systemic infection, drug or poison intoxication (other than alcohol), childbirth, and undiagnosed physical conditions.
2. Nonpsychotic organic brain syndromes (309): This cate-

gory is for patients who have an organic brain syndrome, but who are not psychotic.

J. Mental retardation (310-315): Mental retardation refers to subnormal intellectual functioning which originates during the developmental period and is associated with impairment of either learning and social adjustment or maturation, or both.

1. Borderline mental retardation (310): I.Q. 68-83
2. Mild mental retardation (311): I.Q. 52-67
3. Moderate mental retardation (312): I.Q. 36-51
4. Severe mental retardation (313): I.Q. 20-35
5. Profound mental retardation (314): I.Q. under 20
6. Unspecified mental retardation (315): A classification for patients whose intellectual functioning has not or cannot be evaluated precisely.

Neuroses

I. **Definition:** Maladaptive emotional states resulting from unresolved, unconscious conflicts.

II. **Introduction**
   A. These reactions represent an individual's unsuccessful compromise efforts to deal with underlying primitive needs.
   B. Since anxiety is regarded as the central force in the dynamics of neuroses, the disorders are characterized chiefly by the symptomatic expression of anxiety or the defenses utilized by the ego to control the anxiety.
   C. Freud believed that neuroses resulted from conflict between the ego and the id, in contrast to psychoses which he felt resulted from conflict between the ego and the superego.

III. **General characteristics of neuroses**
   A. Repression is incomplete in the neurotic disorders.
   B. The neurotic compromise is never completely satisfactory since the defenses employed produce symptoms which are experienced as subjective distress and from which the person seeks relief. In addition, the neurotic develops feelings of inferiority and guilt.
   C. Since the form of the neuroses is determined largely by the defenses employed, it represents a defense response.

D. The choice of defenses is in part a product of the individual's character structure and thus is determined by the developmental stage in which fixation occurred or from which the most prominent character traits were derived.
E. Many neurotic disorders have mixed features.
F. The relationships between the subjective symptoms and the underlying conflicts are usually unrecognized by the neurotic.

IV. Comparison with psychoses
A. Psychoses are generally more profound emotional disturbances than neuroses. They usually show more distortion, more disorganization, more disturbed social functioning, and more misinterpretation of external reality than the neuroses.
B. The psychotic's overt behavior is usually more reflective of his underlying disturbed experiences than the neurotic's.
C. The psychotic often lacks recognition that he is ill, whereas the neurotic is usually aware of his distress.
D. Reality is often distorted in the psychotic and is usually unchanged in the neurotic.
E. Freud believed that the psychotic denied reality, whereas the neurotic tried to ignore it.
F. The neurotic is often sensitive to the social world about him whereas the psychotic is not.
G. Conation is usually greatly disturbed in the psychotic.
H. There are certain cases that seem to show characteristics of both. Hence, one might regard abnormal behavior as falling along a spectrum.
I. Any given constellation of psychological factors may lead to the production of neurosis in one person or lead to the development of a psychosis in yet another.

V. Etiology
A. Biologic and genetic factors are not thought to be of any major significance in the cause of neuroses.
B. Social factors are felt by many to play some role. Cultural forces and family interaction seem to play some part in many of the neuroses (as a matter of fact, some present-day psychiatrists feel that the family unit is the proper focus of treatment rather than the individual).
C. Psychogenic factors (both antecedent and concurrent) are regarded by most authorities as the basic etiological factors.
   1. Antecedent factors: Here, the forces operating during the early developmental years seem to have the most important

significance (this would include parental attitudes toward the individual, and the individual's feelings as to whether or not he was accepted and loved).

   a. Disturbances of the child-parent relationship in the earliest years seem particularly significant. For example, a mother who is harsh, overprotective, or inconsistent.

   b. The infant's long period of dependency on his mother seems to be a critical factor.

   c. Thus, the therapist tries to connect the current neurotic symptomatology with some unresolved childhood conflict.

   d. Neurotic traits, such as sleepwalking, enuresis, nail-biting, are often evident in the childhood of adult neurotics.

2. Concurrent factors: Oftentimes in the development of neurotic symptoms, one can see precipitating or immediate causes triggering or initiating the neuroses. These are frequently hostile, sexual, or dependency feelings.

   a. Immediate reality factors may be precipitants rather than causes.

   b. The dehumanizing aspects of modern-day society may represent a psychological threat.

3. Etiology is usually regarded as resulting from a constellation of factors rather than a single cause. Some underlying conflict is usually present and this should be sought out and identified in trying to help the neurotic.

4. Psychogenic etiology is regarded from two major orientations:

   a. Dynamic: This point of view is largely psychoanalytic in orientation and regards anxiety as the central force in the production of neurosis. The various reactions result from the manner in which the ego deals with anxiety.

   b. Physiologic: This regards neuroses as conditioned responses resulting from stressful stimuli with which the individual is unable to cope.

D. A more detailed outline of etiology will be taken up in the sections describing the various clinical types.

VI. **Prevalence:** It seems likely that the neuroses are the conditions most commonly treated by physicians. It is estimated that between one-third and two-thirds of complaints brought to general practitioners and family physicians are essentially functional in origin. Even among physicians who limit their practices to one of the various specialties, the incidence of functional complaints is high.

A. The neurotic reactions are more common among women —perhaps because more repression is expected of them.
B. Neurotic reactions are more common among the upper and middle socioeconomic groups (in contrast to psychotic reactions which are more common in the lower socioeconomic groups).
C. Most of the neurotic reactions are seen during early adult life (from late adolescence to the middle thirties), the period when most people are confronted with the greatest responsibilities and hence show the greatest need for adjustment.

VII. **Classification**
A. Although our present classification is an improvement over previous ones, it still is not fully satisfactory. One of the major reasons for this is that it is based largely on symptomatology rather than on etiological factors, as is true in most other kinds of disease classifications.
B. The neuroses include the following:
1. Anxiety neurosis
2. Phobic neurosis
3. Hysterical neurosis, conversion type
4. Hysterical neurosis, dissociative type
5. Depressive neurosis
6. Obsessive-compulsive neurosis
7. Neurasthenic neurosis (neurasthenia)
8. Depersonalization neurosis (depersonalization syndrome)
9. Hypochondriacal neurosis
10. Other neurosis
C. Each of these reactions will be discussed separately.

ANXIETY NEUROSIS

Synonyms: anxiety reaction, anxiety state, anxiety tension state, stress reaction.

I. **Definition:** Anxiety neurosis is a reaction in which anxiety is the most prominent feature. The uneasiness, apprehension, or fearfulness is experienced directly and is disproportionate to any apparent external cause.

II. **Introduction**
A. Dynamically anxiety neurosis is the simplest type of neurotic reaction.

B. The reader is referred to the chapter on Anxiety for: features, components, patterns, etc.

III. **Symptoms:** In general, the symptoms are similar to those of fear. There is no employment of defense mechanisms to manage or control the anxiety. As noted previously, anxiety can be manifested either as somatic or psychic symptoms.
A. Somatic symptoms: Clinically, the symptoms can be diffusely spread throughout several body systems or may be limited chiefly to one system.
B. Psychic symptoms: The symptoms are subjective and may be difficulty in concentration, uneasiness, apprehension, fear of insanity, or fear of impending disaster.
C. The onset may be acute or insidious.
D. Anxiety attacks result from overstimulation of the autonomic nervous system.
E. Panic is an acute anxiety attack of overwhelming severity which leads to disorganization of ego functions.

IV. **Psychopathology**
A. Anxiety results when some conflict is aroused (or rearoused) either by a weakening of the repressive forces or by strengthening (or reinforcement) of the underlying drive or wish.
B. Thus, repressed conflicts press for reemergence.
C. The symptoms are nonspecific and do not offer any clues as to the underlying etiology. However, the precipitating circumstances and the setting in which attacks occur, especially the first attack, usually give some clues as to the underlying cause.
D. Dynamically, this is the simplest form of neurosis.

V. **Course and prognosis**
A. Usually occurs in attacks; and between attacks the individual may be comfortable, although more commonly he is somewhat tense.
B. If the conflict is not resolved, the individual may utilize one or more of the defense mechanisms and thus develop the picture of one of the other clinical reaction types.
C. Ordinarily, the prognosis in uncomplicated cases is good.
D. Some cases become chronic. In the past, neurasthenia was considered a form of chronic anxiety neurosis. In the present nomenclature, neurasthenic neurosis has a separate classification.
E. An anxiety attack or a panic attack may be the precursor of an

acute undifferentiated schizophrenic reaction (see chapter "Schizophrenia").

VI. Treatment
  A. Short-term supportive psychotherapy is usually indicated. This would include: (1) reassurance and support (not only verbal but attitudinal as well), (2) clarification and education, including pointing out various dynamic and stress factors and supporting various positions and recommendations about changes, and (3) environmental modification, including changing the environment in any way, modifying whatever stresses may be present, and even family therapy.
  B. Insight psychotherapy: Although most psychotherapy aims at giving some insight, certain cases of anxiety neurosis require long-term interpretative psychoanalytically oriented psychotherapy.
  C. Medications: Here reliance is chiefly on the tranquilizers: (1) minor tranquilizers, including meprobamate (Equanil or Miltown); chlordiazepoxide (Librium); diazepam (Valium); (2) major tranquilizers: chlorpromazine (Thorazine); thioridazine (Mellaril); (3) antidepressant medication may be added if depressive symptoms occur.
  D. Deconditioning treatment has been recommended by some. Since much anxiety is a conditioned response, deconditioning has been tried with some success.

VII. Case example: Mrs. J., a thirty-year-old housewife, sought psychiatric treatment because of the following symptoms: irritability, anxiousness, lower abdominal pain, numbness and tingling of her extremities, and marked fearfulness centered chiefly on her health. Although she had been a "nervous" person most of her life, her presenting symptoms had begun three months earlier and occurred in "attacks." During a series of interviews it was learned that the onset of her symptoms dated to the day her sister unexpectedly removed a niece the patient had been caring for in her home. The patient had been caring for the child while the child's mother was hospitalized for delivery of a baby. Two factors in her past history were of dynamic significance: (1) She had been the oldest girl in a large family and cared for the other siblings, especially when her mother was in the hospital having babies; (2) Sterility —she had been unable to conceive after ten years of marriage. Thus, an anxiety reaction is precipitated in a woman desirous of having a family, who in the past had to "give up" children when the mother returned and who again found herself forced to "give up" a child three months earlier.

From a dynamic viewpoint, the symptoms are manifestations of the patient's conflict between her desire for children and her inability to conceive. The fact that she had to "give up" a child three months earlier reactivated the conflict and precipitated the symptoms.

In this case note that the presenting symptoms were both somatic and psychic, were typical of anxiety, and came in attacks. The conflict in this case was relatively superficial.

PHOBIC NEUROSIS

Synonyms: phobic reaction, anxiety hysteria, phobia

  I. Definition: Phobic neurosis is a reaction characterized by a persistent, obsessive fear of a specific object or situation.

  II. Introduction
    A. As a symptom, phobia may occur in a variety of syndromes; for example, phobias that occur in certain other neurotic disorders and phobias that sometimes occur in paranoid or schizophrenic disorders.
    B. Mild phobias are found rather frequently among normal adults; for instance, fear of flying or fear of snakes.
    C. Gross distortion of reality is usually absent.
    D. Phobic reaction was first described by Westphal in 1872.
    E. Freud's case of *Little Hans,* a five-year-old boy who developed a phobia, was described in 1909.

  III. Symptoms
    A. Aside from the phobia itself, the other symptoms are concerned chiefly with ways of avoiding the feared object or situation. This obviously serves to restrict the individual's freedom of action.
    B. The individual has focalized his anxiety, and as long as he can avoid the focalized object or situation, he remains relatively comfortable and free of anxiety.
    C. The type of fear response is in part culturally determined, and as is true in hysterical symptoms, there is a secondary gain factor (for example, fear of airplanes developing in an urban dwelling salesman who has to fly as part of his job).
    D. If confronted with the feared object or situation, the individual develops anxiety (varying from mild uneasiness to marked panic).
    E. The individual recognizes the unreasonableness of the phobia

but is unable to control his behavior or explain why he has the fear.

F. Types of phobias: There are numerous types of phobias since they can develop in relation to almost anything. Clinically, phobias are most commonly seen in relation to the following:
1. Closed spaces (claustrophobia)
2. Open spaces (agoraphobia)
3. Heights (acrophobia)
4. Elevators
5. Dirt
6. Germs
7. Water
8. Crowds
9. Animals
10. Sharp objects, such as knives
11. Harming someone
12. Flying
13. School (this is a phobia found in children and well known to child guidance clinics in the United States. Its origins are rooted in the mother-child dependency relationship).

G. There are many objects and situations that most people fear: snakes, heights, and death.

IV. **Psychopathology** (See repression under "Adjustive Patterns")
A. Essentially, in this disorder, an individual experiences severe, diffuse anxiety which is only incompletely resolved by repression and so there is displacement of the anxiety to an external focus which the individual then tries to avoid (focalizing or binding anxiety).
B. The choice of phobia is sometimes thought to be a matter of fortuitous circumstances, but more commonly it is thought to have a symbolic representation of the underlying impulse or desire. For example, the mother who fears she may harm her youngster unconsciously has some desire to hurt the child; the person who has a marked phobia of dirt may have underlying desires to soil or to be dirty. Some phobias represent the fear of punishment for the underlying unacceptable desire—for example, a fear of knives in one who is tempted to harm himself because of guilt regarding hostility directed toward his spouse.
C. A "phobic partner" or companion is sometimes dynamically involved in this neurosis and is someone who protects the phobic patient. Such a partner is viewed as a symbolic parent helping to satisfy the phobic person's dependency needs.

Many times there seems to be an element of secondary gain for the partner as well.

    D. Sometimes the patient develops counterphobic behavior in which he repeatedly and compulsively confronts himself with the source of anxiety in an attempt to reassure himself that he is in control.

    E. From the above, it is evident that the phobic patient uses the following ego defenses: repression, displacement, symbolization, and avoidance.

V. Course and prognosis

    A. If the conflict is close to consciousness and is dealt with promptly, the prognosis is good.

    B. If the conflict is deep and the reactions are highly disguised or highly symbolic phobias, the prognosis is much more serious.

    C. The presence of compulsive symptoms makes the prognosis less hopeful (in some cases there is little or no difference between this reaction and obsessive-compulsive neurosis).

    D. In some cases, there is a tendency for the phobias to spread. This usually occurs when displacement fails to relieve the anxiety. This further restricts the behavior of the individual.

VI. Treatment

    A. Supportive psychotherapy, including reassurance, suggestion, and emotional support, often is enough to relieve mild phobic responses.

    B. Desensitiziation, deconditioning, or other forms of behavior therapy have been advocated by some. In these treatment techniques, direct attacks are made on the phobic behavior rather than trying to understand the underlying unconscious conflicts.

    C. Insight psychotherapy is usually necessary for the more serious cases.

    D. Sometimes, a combination of a direct attack on the phobia, plus subsequent insight therapy, is the most practical. This is especially true in those cases where the phobia is extremely disruptive of the individual's life.

    E. Group therapy has been helpful, especially when used in conjunction with deconditioning.

    F. Medications, including tranquilizers, are helpful in reducing any associated anxiety.

VII. Case example: Mrs. H., a thirty-five-year-old housewife, consulted a psychiatrist because she feared she would harm her children and

that some harm might come to her husband when he was away at work each day.

Many hours of psychotherapy revealed that in early life she felt rejected by her parents and hoped to get from her husband and marriage what she felt she was denied by her parents. Thus, her own children were viewed as a threat to her relationship with her husband and she felt hostile toward them; she was also hostile toward her husband since she saw him as being a rejecting parent. This hostility was repressed but expressed itself disguised as the phobias that she would harm her children and that her husband might be harmed if he left her. When these conflicts were brought to consciousness, she was subsequently able to resolve them differently and her phobias cleared up.

HYSTERICAL NEUROSIS, CONVERSION TYPE

Synonyms: conversion reaction; conversion hysteria

I. **Definition:** The conversion type of hysterical neurosis is a neurotic disorder in which unconscious conflict is manifested as disguised and symbolic somatic symptoms. That is, the anxiety arising out of some conflictual situation is converted into somatic symptoms in parts of the body innervated by the sensorimotor system (symbolic somatization). Thus, the conflict is reflected as physical symptoms instead of being expressed directly.

II. **Differentiation from malingering:** Hysterical neurosis must be distinguished from *malingering* which is purely conscious.
   A. Definition: Malingering is conscious simulation of illness utilized as an avoidance of an unpleasant or intolerable alternative.
   B. Some behavior may be in part consciously determined and in part unconsciously determined.
   C. Many hysterical patients show histrionic exaggeration of their symptoms, and there is sometimes such an obvious secondary gain factor that one sees them as consciously feigning or simulating disease.
   D. In psychiatry, one should regard malingering as possibly indicative of some serious underlying psychopathology.

III. **Prevalence**
   A. Classical conversion hysteria is less common today than it was at the turn of the century.
   B. However, hysterical *symptoms* are fairly common.

C. Hysterical elements are commonly seen in compensation neurosis.

D. Conversion hysteria is more common among women than among men.

IV. Symptoms
  A. Somatic symptoms
    1. The somatic symptoms can vary widely. Frequently the somatic symptoms simulate organic disease and represent the patient's idea of the disease process. The closeness with which the patient's symptoms approximate the symptoms of an organic disease depends in a large measure on the patient's medical and psychological sophistication.
    2. The somatic symptoms chiefly involve organs which are in contact with the external world (in contrast to the physical symptoms of psychophysiologic reactions which are expressed primarily in organs innervated by the autonomic nervous system).
    3. The distribution of the symptoms is unphysiological and nonanatomical.
    4. Somatic symptoms can be considered under two headings:
      a. Motor symptoms—for example, convulsive states, paralysis, paresis (muscular weakness), aphonia (inability to produce normal speech)
      b. Sensory disturbances—such as analgesia (reduced pain sense), anesthesia (absence of feeling), blindness, deafness, globus hystericus (sensation of lump in throat), and pain (most commonly abdominal)
    5. A hysterical neurosis may prolong or exaggerate symptoms that originally resulted from physical illness.
    6. Hysterical symptoms may develop following an accident. (For discussion of this see the section on "Compensation Neurosis.")
  B. Psychic symptoms:
    1. Mental status evaluation of the person with hysterical neurosis reveals no significant abnormalities.
    2. The outstanding psychological symptom in the hysterical conversion neurosis is the patient's indifference to his illness (la belle indifference). Though he obviously has disabling symptoms, he seems unconcerned and shows no anxiety. This indifference is very striking and is characteristic of this disorder. Occasionally, a person with a hysterical neurosis may seem to enjoy his disability.
    3. Oftentimes the patient shows some of the characteristics of

hysterical personality: excitability, emotional instability, overreactivity, self-dramatization, seductiveness.

V. Psychopathology

A. Essentially, the pschopathology is repression of the conflict with conversion of the anxiety into a somatic symptom which is symbolic of the underlying conflict.

B. At one time it was thought that only sexual conflict produced conversion symptoms. Current theories consider that all types of instinctual impulses may find expression in this manner.

C. The premorbid personality is frequently hysteroid or hysterical (histrionic personality). Such an individual is immature, dependent, emotional, dramatic, exhibitionistic, narcissistic, and manipulative. He goes through the motions of feeling without really experiencing emotion and tends to adopt an overly optimistic, "overly nice," attitude toward life (he has an attitude of "all's right with the world").

D. The precipitating factor may seem trivial but have a special meaning to the person (thus, as in anxiety reaction, it is important to know the setting in which the first hysterical symptoms occur).

E. The choice of symptom may be determined by:
   1. The experience of the organ in relation to the conflict (e.g., paralysis of a hand with which the patient has struck someone in anger).
   2. The suitability of the organ to express the conflicts symbolically (e.g., paralysis of the legs as a defense against meeting a threat; to attack or to flee).
   3. Events may tend to focus the conflict in a specific area (e.g., a tonsillectomy or other type of operative procedure in the throat or neck area may be a precursor to aphonia as an expression of underlying conflict operating at the time of the surgery).

F. In conversion neurosis, both primary (neurotic) gain and secondary gain are observed.
   1. The *primary gain* is the relief of anxiety.
   2. The *secondary gain* is the advantage that accrues to the patient by virtue of his illness. Secondary gain is often a factor in other illnesses, both emotional and physical; however, it is most prominent in the hysterical reactions.

G. Conceptions of psychopathology in conversion neurosis:
   1. Hippocrates: Believed that conversion neurosis resulted from a wandering uterus.

2. In the seventeenth century, hysteria was thought to be due to demoniacal possession.
3. Charcot: Believed it was a genetic reaction which resulted in degeneration of the nervous system. He demonstrated that the hysterical symptoms could be produced and removed by hypnotic suggestion. (He believed that normal people could not be hypnotized.)
4. Janet: Introduced the concept of dissociated mental processes in the subconscious. He demonstrated that automatisms were of unconscious origin.
5. Both Babinski and Bernheim believed that the symptoms resulted from suggestion. Bernheim's extensive work with hypnosis led him to believe that hypnotizability was possible in normal people.
6. Breuer and Freud introduced the concept of repressed conflict with conversion. (Freud believed that the repressed conflict was the oedipal complex.)
7. As noted in the foregoing, most authorities now feel that any highly charged instinct or impulse may be involved.

VI. Course and prognosis

A. In acute cases—where the onset is abrupt and the duration of symptoms has been short—the prognosis is usually favorable with treatment.
B. In those cases where the symptoms have been allowed to remain for a sustained period of time, the prognosis is less hopeful.
  1. In such cases, the *secondary gain factor* operates to decrease the individual's motivation to get well by giving up his symptoms.
  2. However, active treatment in someone who is well motivated is often successful.
C. The relative maturity of the premorbid personality and the intensity of the underlying conflict are factors which must be evaluated in estimating the prognosis.

VII. Treatment

A. Supportive psychotherapy, including emotional support, reassurance, and environmental modification is the most common treatment.
B. Insight psychotherapy: Long-term intensive psychotherapy seems indicated in only a small number of the patients.
C. Various forms of behavior therapy have been tried recently.
D. Medications: Sometimes tranquilizers for relief of accompany-

ing anxiety or antidepressant medication for relief of depressive symptoms is indicated.

VIII. Case example: Mr. J., a forty-five-year-old widower, consulted a psychiatrist because of impotence. His wife had died three years earlier, and immediately after this he had consulted a psychiatrist about mild depressive symptoms. He had been in love with his wife when he first married her, but his affection was replaced by pity after she developed a deforming and disfiguring illness. For several years before her death, he was actually repulsed by her appearance and many times wanted to divorce her, but his conscience would not let him.

Shortly before he had presented himself complaining of impotence, a woman whom he had been dating for a few months began to pressure him for a marriage proposal. After three interviews he was able to bring to light the two conflicts which were operative in his impotence: (1) his present relationship rearoused his repressed guilt about his rejection of his wife and (2) he really felt hostile toward the woman he was currently dating for aggressively seeking marriage with him. The symptom thus served a twofold purpose: (1) punishment for his guilt about his wife and (2) hostile expression toward the woman he was dating.

HYSTERICAL NEUROSIS, DISSOCIATIVE TYPE

Synonym: dissociative reaction

I. Definition: A reaction in which there is an automatic unconscious separation, splitting-off, or detachment of certain functions or parts of the personality.

II. Introduction
  A. This is gross personality disorganization which is neurotic in character. However, at times the reaction may be so diffuse as to appear psychotic.
  B. In this reaction, there are alterations in the patient's state of consciousness or in his identity.
  C. The dissociation produces a demonstrable change in a person's behavior, feelings, or thoughts.

III. Psychopathology
  A. Essentially this is the mechanism of dissociation—that is, the unconscious detachment of certain behavior or personality activities from the normal or usual conscious behavior patterns

of an individual which then usually function alone (compart-mentalization).

B. It is a more massive type of forgetting than is seen in simple repression.

C. The ego is protecting itself against something that is critically dangerous and defending itself against overwhelming anxiety that develops because of an emotional bind.

D. Although the dissociation is handicapping, it does relieve the individual's anxiety.

E. Dissociation is also symbolic and may have more than one meaning to the patient.

F. Primary gain (relief of anxiety) and secondary gain (advantage that accrues to the patient by virtue of his reaction) are evident in this condition (similar to hysterical neurosis, conversion type in this regard).

G. Premorbid personality is said to show immaturity, egocentricity, and the presence of some type of episodic emotional disturbance during early life. Still others are said to show hysteroid, schizoid, or passive characteristics.

IV. **Types** (See also discussion of Dissociation in the chapter on "Adjustive Patterns")

A. Amnesia: Pathological loss of memory (this type of amnesia must be distinguished from the amnesia associated with organic brain damage).

1. It is more than a mere forgetting. Rather, it is an active "blotting out" of consciousness containing conflictual material.

2. It is most often a response to intense feelings such as terror, anger, or guilt.

3. Ordinarily it has a sudden onset and is of brief duration.

4. The individual usually has an attitude of indifference to his memory loss (similar to the indifference in conversion reactions).

5. Case example: Mrs. H., a forty-two-year-old housewife, entered the hospital complaining of several brief periods of memory loss. History revealed that the onset of these episodes coincided with the time that she first learned her husband was going out with another woman and that subsequent episodes usually followed some incident in which she was reminded of the "other woman."

B. Fugue: A personality dissociation characterized by memory loss and flight from the immediate environment.

1. During this changed state of consciousness, the individual

operates on his unconscious strivings. In the fugue, the individual often performs complicated activities and permits himself to follow the unconscious feelings which his conscience ordinarily restrains him from doing. In a sense, the fugue state permits him to do a certain amount of "acting out."

2. In addition, the individual sometimes "loses" his identity by "forgetting" his name, and at other times, he "changes" his identity by assuming a different name.

3. Oftentimes he may appear quite normal to observers.

4. Amnesia may follow the termination of the fugue.

5. Case example: J. R., a twenty-five-year-old soldier, was admitted to the prison ward of a military hospital accused of desertion. History revealed he had served with distinction in combat and was twice wounded. Following his second wound, he was evacuated to the United States mainland for further treatment. After a brief period at one hospital, the medical staff decided he could be managed best at another hospital several hundred miles away and placed him on a train for that destination. The man never arrived at the second hospital, but six months later was discovered in another section of the country living the life of a civilian under an assumed name. He was unable to identify himself correctly and could not account for his activities during the entire six-month period. His real identity was established only through his fingerprints.

C. Dissociative experiences related to sleep including somnambulism and sleeptalking.

D. Ganser syndrome (sometimes called the nonsense syndrome or prison psychosis): It is commonly employed by those who seek to mislead others regarding their true emotional state.

1. It occurs chiefly in prisoners who are confined.

2. It is characterized by childish, ludicrous behavior.

3. The individual's replies or responses are approximate (hence, it is sometimes called "the syndrome of approximate answers").

4. It is not a form of malingering.

E. Automatism: Unconscious automatic and apparently unguided symbolic behavior, as for example, automatic handwriting.

F. Multiple personality (dual personality): The unconscious adoption of two or more different personalities which are separate and compartmentalized. Generally, the primary character is proper and moral while the secondary personality is hedonistic and impulse-ridden.

G. Amok, berserk, Arctic madness, and others: These are all acute outbursts of violence that occur in various cultures. They are usually considered hysterical dissociative reactions, although they might also be classed as depersonalization reactions.

V. Course and prognosis

A. The course and prognosis depend upon the patient's motivation to get well, his ego-strength, the duration of the reaction, and the strength of the secondary gain factor.

B. In general those dissociative episodes which have an acute onset have a good immediate prognosis.

C. Those in which there is a close relationship between some environmental factor and onset have a good prognosis when removed from the threatening environment.

D. The long-term prognosis in some cases is only fair.

E. The symptoms of any of these particular dissociative phenomenon usually increase when the patient is confronted with mounting anxiety.

VI. Treatment

A. The treatment should be dynamic or psychoanalytically oriented psychotherapy.

B. See section on hysterical neurosis, conversion type, for additional treatment recommendations.

DEPERSONALIZATION NEUROSIS (DEPERSONALIZATION SYNDROME)

I. **Definition:** A disorder of affect in which the person has feelings of unreality, altered personality, or altered identity. He may deny his own existence or that of his environment.

II. Introduction

A. The syndrome is dominated by a feeling of unreality and of estrangement from the self, body, or surroundings. This diagnosis should not be employed if the condition is part of some other mental disorder. A brief experience of depersonalization is not necessarily a symptom of illness (DSM-II).

B. There are certain depersonalization experiences which are common and not considered pathological. For example, hypnagogic hallucinations (the mental images that occur just before sleep) and hypnopompic hallucinations (images seen in dreams which persist on awakening). These are both found in healthy people.

III. Types

A. Trance-states and trancelike states: A trance-state is a psychological stupor characterized by immobility and unresponsiveness to the environment. It usually has a sudden onset and amnesia. A trancelike state is a similar experience that is ordinarily induced in a "normal individual" after prolonged and unusual concentration on a task or object.

B. Feelings of unreality (a feeling that one is unreal) and feelings of derealization (feeling that the environment has changed) and depersonalization (a sense of estrangement from one's self).

C. *Déjà vu:* A subjective sensation that an experience which really is happening for the first time occurred on a previous occasion. Occurs in normal people, neurotic reaction, psychotic reaction, and organic brain syndromes.

D. Feelings of estrangement (a sense of detachment from people, the environment or concepts); and paramnesia (distortion or falsification of memory in which the individual confuses reality and fantasy).

E. Fascination (or fixation): A trancelike state in an individual who is compelled to focus on a given object for long periods of time (e.g., fliers).

F. Cosmic consciousness or illumination: A fabulous sense of joy or well-being. Sometimes produced from hallucinogenic drugs.

IV. Psychopathology: See hysterical neurosis, dissociative type

V. Course and Prognosis: See hysterical neurosis, dissociative type

VI. Treatment: See hysterical neurosis, dissociative type

DEPRESSIVE NEUROSIS

Synonyms: reactive depressive; depressive reaction; neurotic depression

I. **Although depressive neurosis** is properly classified as one of the neurotic disorders, it seems more appropriate to consider this in the section on affective disorders.

OBSESSIVE-COMPULSIVE NEUROSIS

Synonyms: obsessive-compulsive reaction; obsessional neurosis; obsessive-ruminative state; psychasthenia (an obsolete term originally introduced by Janet); anancastic reactions.

I. **Definition:** Obsessive-compulsive neurosis is characterized by obsessions (persistent, recurring ideas or impulses that remain in consciousness despite their irrationality) and compulsions (illogical, repetitive, and undesired urges to perform acts which are against the person's ordinary wishes).

II. **Features of this neurosis include**
   A. The obsessive ideas persistently intrude themselves into the patient's consciousness.
   B. The obsessions and the compulsions are discomforting (ego-alien).
   C. The patient recognizes the unreasonableness and absurdity of the obsessions and compulsions, but is unable to control them (note the resemblance to phobic reactions).
   D. He feels a strong need to resist the obsessions and compulsions.

III. **Prevalence**
   A. Fleeting obsessions or compulsions are more or less universal.
   B. Obsessive-compulsive neurosis constitutes about 5 percent of neurotic reactions.
   C. The incidence may be somewhat higher because people with this disorder often conceal their symptoms and avoid consulting a physician about them.
   D. Obsessive-compulsive traits are not uncommon in children and adolescents.

IV. **Symptoms**
   A. These symptoms may take many forms. Doubt and vacillation are very prominent.
   B. Obsessions: These recurring ideas or impulses can be about anything. Common themes are as follows:
      1. Violence—for example, homicidal thoughts about a spouse or child
      2. Sexuality
      3. Obscenities
      4. Religion or religious subjects (scrupulosity)
      5. Sometimes the ideas may be quite neutral or indifferent.

(The term *obsessive-ruminative state* is sometimes given to this group.)

C. Compulsions: These are recurrent, compelling acts which develop in an attempt to relieve obsessions or fears. They are of two types: (1) those that are a reaction to or an attempt to control the underlying obsession and (2) those that give direct expression to the underlying obsessive urges—these are rare, and are similar to counterphobic measures in phobic reactions. Common themes of compulsions are:

   1. Contamination—for example, handwashing rituals which develop as a means of relieving fears of, or obsessions about, dirt or germs.

   2. Self-mutilation—for example, self-inflicted excoriations as a compulsive punishment for guilt over masturbation.

D. As can be noted from the foregoing, the obsessions are mostly asocial in nature and the compulsions are mostly "caricatures of morality." In fully developed cases there is a 50-50 ratio between the obsessions and compulsions. Such a state of dynamic equilibrium explains the underlying indecision, uncertainty, and ambivalence found in these patients.

E. Sometimes the compulsive behavior becomes extremely elaborate and the individual may feel compelled to carry out certain rituals, such as counting, touching, or handwashing.

F. In some cases the symptoms are less specific, but rather are manifested as compulsive and ritualistic qualities in all of the individual's behavior. (E.g., the individual who carries out certain rituals on arising in the morning, or who dresses according to a certain pattern, or who performs daily tasks and duties according to a fixed and exact sequence.)

G. In obsessive-ruminative states there is a central rumination about some topic, often of a religious or philosophical nature. The matter is repeatedly meditated upon, giving consideration to the pros and cons and imponderables, etc., but no definite decisions are ever reached; rather, the matter remains inconclusive.

H. Because the patient is often embarrassed about his compulsions and rituals, he may go to great lengths to disguise them from others. If the compulsions become more severe or chronic, his ability to hide the acts becomes progressively less successful.

I. Other features: It is said that a large number of obsessive-compulsive neurotics remain unmarried. Some studies indicate that the reaction is more common among people in the upper socioeconomic class and those of high IQ. There apparently are no sex differences.

V. Psychopathology: This reaction is dynamically much more complicated than any of the other neuroses.

A. Repression for some reason is unsuccessful (or only incompletely successful) and the individual makes use of other defenses to reinforce the repression. These subsequent defenses are:

1. Isolation: The separation of an unacceptable impulse, act, or idea from its memory origin, thereby removing the emotional charge associated with the original memory.
   a. For example, violent or unacceptable ideas may be present but can be accepted because they are separated from the rest of the mental content.
   b. This mechanism is the basis of many compulsive rituals.
   c. Typically, the obsessive-compulsive neurotic remains emotionally aloof from highly charged situations.

2. Reaction formation: The direction of overt behavior or attitudes in precisely the opposite direction of the individual's underlying, unacceptable impulses (the underlying impulses may be conscious or unconscious).
   a. For example, the patient who wants to be dirty develops washing rituals as a defense; oversolicitousness and overprotectiveness may be an attempt to hide hostile and rejecting feelings.
   b. Submissiveness, excessive amiability, or excessive concern may be reaction formation against underlying hostility, aggression, or death wishes.
   c. Compulsive meticulousness may cover up strong soiling impulses.
   d. Reaction formation results in the development of character traits more often than symptoms.

3. Undoing: A primitive defense mechanism in which some unacceptable past behavior is symbolically acted out in reverse, usually repetitiously (symbolic atonement).
   a. It is the treating of an experience as if it never occurred.
   b. It is closely related to reaction formation (magical expiation).
   c. Examples:
      (1) Handwashing may represent expiation for various types of antisocial or asocial behavior.
      (2) Initially felt hostility toward a person may be undone by later ingratiating behavior.

4. Displacement: The redirection of an emotion from the original object to a more acceptable substitute object.
   a. Feelings of hostility initially felt toward parents may be transferred to parent surrogates or other authority figures.
   b. Handwashing may result from the displacement of feelings concerning moral uncleanness to dirt which must be continually cleansed away.
B. Ambivalence (the coexistence of two opposing feelings toward the same individual or object) is very prominent in obsessive-compulsive neurotics. Feelings often involve love and hate. Ambivalence is also evident in the doing-undoing behavior described above.
C. Premorbid personality: Typically the individuals who develop this type of reaction have obsessional characteristics. That is, they are rigid, restricted, orderly, meticulous, cautious, deliberate, conscientious, and dependable. The person who possesses such compulsive qualities is also referred to as an *anankastic personality,* or *anal character* (such an individual needs to feel in control of himself and his environment). The presence of these traits does not constitute abnormality. Most of the people who have obsessive-compulsive traits in their personality makeup do not become obsessive-compulsive neurotics.
   1. According to psychoanalytic theory, such anal qualities develop in the infant during the period of toilet-training (anal phase of infantile sexuality). The development of obsessive-compulsive neurosis represents fixation at, or regression to, this anal phase of development—a period when the superego is harsh, demanding, and punitive.
   2. According to learning theory, obsessions are conditioned stimulus responses to anxiety, and compulsions are behavioral patterns which reduce the anxiety.
D. The function of the compulsive act is to allay and bind anxiety.
E. The acts are symbolic.
F. Unlike the patient who has conversion neurosis, the patient who has obsessive-compulsive neurosis is uncomfortable and is dealing more actively with his conflict.

VI. Course and prognosis
A. The onset may occur at any period of life but commonly begins in adolescence. This is probably because this is a period when there is increased sexual awareness, conflict about dependency and independency, etc.

B. Some are transitory and relatively circumscribed episodes. These frequently have a good prognosis with psychotherapy.

C. Unfortunately, many of these reactions have a tendency to become chronic and often follow a remitting course. As such they are often resistant to treatment.

D. Obsessive-compulsive traits found in childhood often clear up or respond promptly to treatment.

E. In general, the prognosis is more favorable in those cases where:
1. The symptoms are of short duration.
2. Environmental stress factors are prominent.
3. If there is good environment to return to following treatment.
4. If interpersonal relationships are good.

VII. **Treatment**
A. Psychotherapy
1. Intensive psychoanalytically oriented psychotherapy at one time was thought to be the treatment of choice. However, it would now appear that only a small number of people with this disorder will respond to this kind of treatment.
2. Supportive psychotherapy is often helpful for many cases. However, it should be kept in mind that responses to psychotherapy often will last only a matter of hours and then the individual's doubts, etc., recur.

B. Behavioral therapy has been tried recently. In this, the underlying complexities of the neurosis are largely ignored and attempts are made to focus on the person's external behavior (similar to behavioral treatment attempts in phobic neurosis).

C. Medications: Sometimes tranquilizers and antidepressant medications are useful in relieving some of the symptoms that accompany obsessive-compulsive neurosis, but none of the known psychotropic drugs relieves the underlying obsessive-compulsive disorder.

D. Hospitalization may be indicated when ritualistic behavior becomes intense.

E. Somatic therapy:
1. Electroshock therapy has been used, often with disappointing results.
2. Prefrontal leukotomy has been performed in some who have chronic crippling disorders.

VIII. **Case example:** Mrs. B., a thirty-three-year-old housewife, consulted a psychiatrist complaining of fear of germs and dirt, obsessions about religious ideas, and obsessions about the number 3. These symptoms had begun about three months earlier, following the birth of her second child. She had had a similar episode five years earlier after her first child was born. This lasted about six months and finally cleared up under counselling with her pastor.

She was a bright person who was always orderly, methodical, conscientious, and dependable. As a child she was overly concerned with the "normal" compulsions that children have, such as counting the pickets in fences, avoiding the cracks in sidewalks, etc. At age ten she became obsessed with the idea that she would die on a certain Tuesday in October.

With her present episode she had developed a number of compulsions in response to her fears and obsessions. For example, she washed her hands repeatedly and relaundered clothes because of her fear of germs and dirt, and she avoided reading automobile license plates and house numbers because she wished to avoid the number 3. After several weeks in the hospital she improved enough so that she was able to carry on with her housework, although she was still troubled somewhat by her symptoms.

In this case, note the previous compulsive personality and the typical obsessions and compulsions. In view of her compulsive personality and incomplete response to hospital treatment, one must be very cautious in prognosticating her future.

NEURASTHENIC NEUROSIS (NEURASTHENIA)

Synonyms: nervous exhaustion; in the past, some of the neurasthenic disorders were considered to be chronic anxiety neuroses or special types of depressive neuroses.

   I. **Definition:** A neurosis characterized by symptoms of weakness, marked fatigability, overwhelming exhaustion, poor concentration, feelings of inadequacy, and an exaggerated attention to bodily organs and functions.

  II. **Introduction**
    A. Beard originally introduced the concept of "nervous exhaustion" in 1867 and viewed the physical change in the nerves as similar to a battery which has lost its charge.
    B. As originally defined, it was considered the forerunner of other more severe nervous disorders such as hysteria and epilepsy.

C. S. Weir Mitchell developed the "Rest Cure" for this condition ("Dr. Diet and Dr. Quiet") as a means of restoring the nerves to their previous state.
D. Whereas Beard believed that fatique and overwork were causal factors in this condition, Bleuler believed that work was helpful in treating it.
E. Current etiological concepts emphasize the role of psychogenic factors.

III. Prevalence
A. Fatigue and tiredness are fairly common symptoms.
B. However, neurasthenia is not a common clinical diagnosis today.

IV. Symptoms
A. There are a wide variety of symptoms in this disorder.
B. Chronic overwhelming exhaustion, weakness, fatigability, multiple aches, pains, strange physical sensations, and an exaggerated attention to bodily organs and functions.
C. The individual often feels exhausted on awakening in the morning but feels better as the day progresses. Exertion of any type seems difficult for him.
D. Other physical symptoms, including gastrointestinal, cardiovascular, genitourinary, etc., may be important.
E. Symptoms of depression and anxiety are often present. Sleep disturbance (particularly insomnia) and irritability are common.
F. A person who has this disorder may have had parents who had somatic illnesses or somatic symptoms of marked severity. Thus, the individual's neurasthenia may be in part an identification.
G. Women with neurasthenia often have dysmenorrhea.

V. Psychopathology
A. Generally, it develops in an individual who has an asthenic personality (such a behavior pattern is characterized by easy fatigability, low energy level, lack of enthusiasm, marked incapacity for enjoyment, and oversensitivity to physical and emotional stress).
B. In general, neurasthenia is seen as a reaction to any kind of conflictual situation (see introductory comments on neuroses at the beginning of this chapter). Thus, it might be considered a reaction to sexual conflict; a reaction to repressed hostility; a disappointment reaction; or a failure reaction, etc.

VI. Course and prognosis: The course is usually a chronic one although it may be intermittent.

VII. Treatment
   A. No specific treatment has been very effective.
   B. Psychotherapy: Unfortunately this has had limited value, but its best results have been in early cases.
   C. The person who is suspected of having this kind of reaction should have careful physical and laboratory examinations to rule out any underlying physical disease.
   D. Medications: Various drugs have been prescribed for symptomatic relief. Included in these are tranquilizers for any anxiety symptoms; antidepressants for any depressive features, etc. Oftentimes, drugs have only temporary effects.
   E. Occasionally, environmental modification is helpful.

VIII. Case example: A thirty-three-year-old Roman Catholic nun who taught junior high school sought psychiatric consultation because of fatigue. She reported that she lacked stamina and felt inadequate. Even as a child she experienced tiredness and exhaustion. At the age of twenty-five she had been hospitalized for two weeks because of exhaustion secondary to tension. She required much rest and at times had even "slept the clock around." Physical and laboratory examinations by her personal physician on a number of occasions were unrevealing.

HYPOCHONDRIACAL NEUROSIS

Synonyms: hypochondriasis; in the past some of the anxiety reactions and some of the psychophysiologic disorders were included under this term.

   I. Definition: A neurosis characterized by persistent and obsessive preoccupation with physical or emotional health, and accompanied by various somatic symptoms without demonstrated organic cause.

   II. Introduction
   A. The hypochondriac is painfully aware of sensations that most people ignore. In general, he exaggerates their intensity and importance.
   B. The term derives from the term for the subcostal abdominal region, the hypochondrium, which at one time was believed to be the seat of origin of the disorder.
   C. It is now presumed to be of psychogenic origin.
   D. The hypochondriac's somatic preoccupation precludes his

being able to concern himself with underlying feelings or conflicts.

III. Symptoms
A. As noted in the foregoing, this type of neurotic is aware of physical sensations that most others disregard.
B. Sometimes the somatic preoccupation is really an obsessional symptom, and may represent displacement of anxiety onto the body itself.
C. Sometimes the hypochondriacal symptoms are vague and at other times they are organ-centered.

IV. Psychopathology
A. For psychopathological considerations, see section on neurasthenic neuroses.
B. Also, see introductory section on the neuroses.

V. Treatment
A. See section on neurasthenic neuroses.
B. In general, psychotherapy has had limited value.
C. Careful physical evaluation is necessary to make sure that a person's somatic symptoms do not in fact represent physical disease. Also, it is important to remember that a hypochondriacal person can develop serious physical disease.

VI. Case example: A sixty-year-old married woman was referred for psychiatric treatment by her personal physician because of symptoms of nausea, anorexia, nervousness, and numerous other physical symptoms related to her gastrointestinal tract. These had been present for at least ten years. She gave a history of reacting to most stressful situations with various somatic symptoms: shakiness, leg aches, headache, etc. Although she had a proven peptic ulcer in the past, her own physician was satisfied from his repeated physical evaluation of her that none of her somatic symptoms were due to organic disease.

OTHER NEUROSES

I. **This classification** is reserved for those neurotic disorders which cannot be classified elsewhere.

II. **It includes** such reactions as writer's cramp, and other occupational neuroses.

COMPENSATION NEUROSIS

Synonyms: accident neurosis; occupational neurosis (occupational syndrome); traumatic neurosis (this latter term includes neuroses in which the trauma is of psychological as well as physical origin).

I. **Definition:** Compensation neurosis is a neurotic reaction in which secondary gain factors are conspicuous. The secondary gain may be any external benefit which is derived from the illness; for example, disability benefits, financial gain, or personal attention. *Traumatic neurosis:* A term which includes combat, occupational, and compensation reactions.

   A. Refers to a tendency to maintain those symptoms which originally arose in occupational or accident settings as a defense against loss of any derived secondary gains.

   B. It includes reactions which are commonly related to occupational factors such as writer's cramp or miner's nystagmus.

II. **Introduction**

   A. Sometimes these reactions are considered as types of hysterical neurosis, conversion type since conversion symptoms are often quite prominent.

   B. However, many compensation neuroses have symptoms other than hysteria, including anxiety, pain, depression, etc.

   C. It is not an official diagnosis in the *Diagnostic and Statistical Manual* (DSM-II) but is sometimes classified under the category "Other Neuroses" (300.8).

III. **Symptoms**

   A. The symptom pictures in these conditions vary; frequently there are somatic symptoms, pain which limits or incapacitates the individual, anxiety, depression, sleeplessness, irritability, etc. In addition, the patient is often loquaciously descriptive of his feelings and symptoms. However, although he complains a good bit about his symptoms, he rarely asks how he can be rid of them.

   B. Sometimes the serious symptoms of which the patient complains and which are the disabling feature do not appear until some period after the accident. That is, there is an incubation period between the injury and the appearance of the neurotic symptomatology. At other times, the serious symptoms do not appear until he has made an attempt to return to his job.

C. The symptom picture is not essentially different from other neuroses except in the matter of involvement of compensation.

D. The symptoms have sometimes been more permanently fixed by the tendency to repeated examinations and overtreatment.

IV. Psychopathology

A. At one time it was thought that the principal, if not the exclusive, etiological determinant in this kind of reaction was the desire for adequate compensation. Recent studies have shown that other factors are operative. For example, some authors have commented on the presence of paranoid traits, the underlying need for attention, underlying job dissatisfaction, etc.

B. Extensive investigations into the accident process by Hirshfeld and Behan have brought to light the following important psychological factors:

1. The prodromal period, preceding the accident or moment of harm, was identical with the postdromal period except for the actual injury and physical impairment. One of the principal characteristics of the prodrome was that the patient gave repeated evidences of depression and anxiety prior to the accident. In the postdromal period, the depression had changed to anger following the injury. They also observed that most compensation cases represent very little, if any, actual physical harm. Thus, the accident or moment of harm changed an unacceptable disability into one that was acceptable or desirable for the patient.

This can be diagramed as:

Prodrome→ Moment of Harm → Postdrome

2. They also described certain personality types associated with accident victims. These were:
   a. Dependent personalities
   b. Punishment seekers (hari-kiri personalities)
   c. Passive-resisters (Ghandi syndrome)
   d. Poorly identified personalities
   e. Depressive personalities
   f. Psychotic personalities

3. They also found that best treatment results of these neurotic reactions were obtained by broadly based physicians rather than specialists, such as psychiatrists.

C. Social custom and public opinion have tended to encourage this problem.

D. Workmen's Compensation Acts and industrial and automobile accident insurance programs have increased the incidence of compensation neurosis.

E. Litigation helps to maintain the individual's focus on his injury, but it should be kept in mind that settlement with the resultant termination of litigation often does not relieve the symptoms of compensation neurosis. The present trend of social legislation in relation to occupation indicates that other psychiatric disabilities arising out of work stress of a more general nature are also being considered work-related and the company or its insurance carrier is being held responsible.

V. **Treatment**

A. The main emphasis in any treatment regime should be on prevention. This means that a person who is injured in relationship to his occupation or an accident should be given very careful, thorough evaluation (examination should not be just limited to the area with symptoms).

B. Generally, a supportive, optimistic, and reassuring approach in dealing with people who have work-related or accident-related problems will diminish the chances of developing neurotic disability.

C. Formal psychiatric treatment, such as psychotherapy or somatic therapies, are usually ineffective when tried, mostly because the cases that are referred for psychiatric treatment are chronic and firmly fixed (including the locking-in of the patient's hostility).

D. Various kinds of medications, including tranquilizers, are sometimes helpful in alleviating some of the distressing symptoms.

REFERENCES

Bosselman, B. C. *Neurosis and Psychosis.* 3rd ed. Springfield, Illinois: Charles C. Thomas Publishers, 1964, chap. II, III, IV, V.

Freedman, A. M.; Kaplan, H. I.; and Sadock, B. J. *Modern Synopsis of Comprehensive Textbook of Psychiatry.* Baltimore: Williams & Wilkins, 1972, chap. XIX.

Kolb, L. C. *Modern Clinical Psychiatry.* 8th ed. Philadelphia: W. B. Saunders Company, 1973, chap. XXIV.

I find, by experience, that the mind and the
  body are more than married,
For they are most intimately united;
And when the one suffers, the other
  sympathizes.

Lord Chesterfield (Philip T.
Stanhope), 1694-1773

Psychophysiologic Disorders

Synonyms: psychosomatic disorders; functional disorders; organ neuroses

I. **Definition:** Psychophysiologic disorders are a group of reactions characterized by somatic symptoms that result from emotional factors and involve organ systems usually innervated by the autonomic nervous system (which is not under voluntary control).

II. **Introduction**
  A. The physiological changes involved are those that usually accompany emotional response, but in the psychophsiologic reactions, the changes are more intense, more sustained, and involve a single organ system.
    1. Symptoms are thus physiological rather than symbolic as is true in conversion neurosis. Examples of physical symptoms from emotional causes: tachycardia from anger; tears from grief; constipation from depression; diarrhea from anxiety.
    2. Presumably, if such physiological expression of affect continues over a long period of time, structural changes may result in the body.
  B. Psychophysiologic expression of anxiety is seen to some degree in all humans, under some circumstances. Thus, it is important

to keep in mind that psychophysiologic responses are present to some degree in all illness. However, it is only in the so-called "psychosomatic" conditions that the individual is reacting to unconscious stress from prior events. (The responses seen in people with physical illness represent responses to the current situation and are identifiable.)

C. Emotional factors play a major, but not necessarily an exclusive, etiologic role.

D. Actually, to speak of the psyche and the soma as if they were two separate entities is an artificiality, since the two are really inseparable. Thus, in a broad sense, all illness is "psychosomatic" since most organic illnesses have emotional aspects and most emotional illnesses have physical components.

E. Psychophysiologic medicine (psychosomatic medicine) is concerned with the following:

1. Physical symptoms from emotional causes, as for example, palpitation, tachycardia, and precordial distress as manifestations of anxiety neurosis; or paresis (muscle weakness) of an extremity as a conversion phenomenon.

2. Physical disease from causes that were presumed to be initally emotional, as for example, essential hypertension; peptic ulcer; migraine headaches.

3. Organic disease in which certain symptoms arise from emotional factors, as for example, tachycardia and palpitation occurring in a person with rheumatic heart disease, not as a result of cardiac dysfunction per se but as a manifestation of anxiety about the amount of feared physical disability.

F. Strictly speaking, psychophysiologic disorders do not include the psychological reactions to physical illness. However, it is common for many clinicians to regard such reactions as "psychosomatic" problems.

G. In the past, there were three main schools of thought regarding the specificity of conflict in the psychophysiologic disorders:

1. The "specificity" model: The psychological factors which produce a particular type of disorder were regarded as specific and symbolic.

2. The "nonspecific" model: Many different psychological factors may produce a given disorder. The nature of the response depends upon acquired vulnerability of the organ and upon constitutional factors.

3. "Individual response specificity": A specific constellation of

psychological factors plus a somatic local vulnerability produce a particular psychophysiologic disorder. (This theory has taken into account both local vulnerability and psychogenic specificity.)

4. No one theory has received unanimous acceptance by psychosomatic investigators.
5. Most authorities would agree that specific psychophysiologic disorders are not related to specific psychological conflict.

III. Current theories regarding etiology

A. The underlying etiological factors in psychophysiologic reactions are similar to those for the neuroses.

Thus, they are similar to those neurotic reactions in which the somatic reflections are expressed in one or more body systems; for example, the tachycardia and palpitation in anxiety neurosis; the anorexia and constipation in depressive neurosis.

B. Psychophysiologic disorders, like most other aspects of human behavior, can be considered to be overdetermined; that is, they have multiple causations.

C. Experiential factors may play a conditioning role.

D. Whether the particular body system involved is due to an unconscious symbolism or to latent vulnerability is not really known at this point.

E. A given psychophysiologic response may be due to any one of a number of emotions; for example, diarrhea may be associated with rage, anxiousness, or unmet dependency needs.

F. The importance of emotions in any particular case of psychophysiologic reaction varies (e.g., peptic ulcer under psychophysiologic gastrointestinal disorders).

G. Some authorities feel that the psychophysiologic reactions are most commonly seen during the middle-age period.

H. These disorders constitute about one-fifth of the case load of family physicians.

IV. Types of psychophysiologic disorders

A. Psychophysiologic gastrointestinal disorder
B. Psychophysiologic cardiovascular disorder
C. Psychophysiologic respiratory disorder
D. Psychophysiologic genitourinary disorder
E. Psychophysiologic musculoskeletal disorder
F. Psychophysiologic skin disorder
G. Psychophysiologic endocrine disorder
H. Psychophysiologic hemic and lymphatic disorder

I. Psychophysiologic disorder of organ of special sense

J. Psychophysiologic disorder of other type

V. Psychophysiologic gastrointestinal disorders

A. From early life, food is associated with feelings of security, attention, and love. Conflicts centering around these emotions may contribute to gastrointestinal disturbances.

B. The role of psychogenic factors in some of the gastrointestinal reactions seems well accepted.

C. Disorders of the upper gastrointestinal tract are often associated with oral character structure, whereas diseases of the lower gastrointestinal system are often associated with anal character structure.

D. Specific reactions

1. Obesity

   a. With rare exceptions, obesity results from overeating.

   b. Many obese individuals overeat when they are emotionally upset. Obese persons are more likely to manifest neurotic traits and symptoms than are people of normal weight.

   c. Overeating is a symptom of underlying emotional problems and may be used to:

      (1) Allay anxiety,

      (2) Obtain gratification, or

      (3) Express hostility.

   d. The overeater is <u>orally fixate</u>d and hence resorts to food in an attempt to allay his anxiety. The obese person grows dependent on food much as the addict becomes dependent on drugs.

   e. The overeater turns to food for gratification when he is unhappy or inclined to self-pity.

   f. Obesity is sometimes regarded as an affect equivalent and results from unfullfilled needs for love. In a sense, food is used as a tranquilizer.

   g. In certain cases obesity may represent a desire to be unattractive; this is usually accompanied by fear of sexuality.

   h. Patterns of overeating vary. Included are the "binge" type (sudden compulsive ingestion of large amounts of food in a short period of time) and night-eating (morning anorexia, evening hyperphagia, and insomnia).

   i. Although the fat person is often outwardly jovial and congenial, underlying (repressed) hostility is often a cause for overeating.

    j. Treatment by dietary management without giving attention to the underlying psychopathology is usually not successful.

    k. Group therapy has been used with some success for obese persons, including groups that are not under professional direction (similar to group therapy with the alcoholics).

2. Anorexia nervosa

    a. Definition: A syndrome found in young people, characterized by marked, prolonged appetite loss with accompanying marked weight loss (psychogenic malnutrition).

    b. It was assumed at one time that only females suffered from this disturbance, but about 10 percent of the cases are males.

    c. Often the individual seems unusually active for the amount of appetite loss and weight loss.

    d. Amenorrhea is usual in females.

    e. Usually no other evidences of starvation are found.

    f. Presumably results from oral conflicts and the individual's rejection of oral propensities (reaction formation to the dependency needs).

    g. Mentally, patients are found to be depressed, hysterical, obsessive-compulsive, or schizophrenic.

    h. It is important to differentiate this condition from endocrine and other organic illnesses that produce malnutrition, loss of appetite, and weight loss.

    i. Treatment must include a combined medical and psychiatric approach. The treatment must be individualized to cope with the underlying psychopathology. Patients are often refractory to treatment.

    j. Oftentimes histories of such individuals indicate periods of anorexia and weight loss alternating with periods of bulimia (pathologically increased hunger) and obesity.

3. Peptic ulcer

    a. Opinions regarding the cause of peptic ulcer vary from those of persons who regard ulcer formation as a strictly organic process to those who believe the etiology is almost exclusively psychological.

    b. Peptic ulcer is regarded as a disease of civilization and is more prevalent in urban areas and is much more common among men than women.

c. Experimental observations (H. G. Wolfe and S. Wolf) indicate that prolonged emotional tension plus an external irritant on a sensitized stomach may result in ulcer formation.

d. Current theories regard peptic ulcer formation as resulting from emotional conflict plus the proper hypersecreting type of gastric mucosa (based on gastric fistula studies in animals and humans also).

e. Psychopathological aspects
   (1) Franz Alexander: In 1934 described what he regarded as the conflict between oral-receptive tendencies (the wish to be taken care of) and a striving for independence. The oral tendencies and fantasies produced continuous gastric secretion which he believed lead to ulcer formation.
   (2) A. J. Sullivan and T. E. McKell: Believed Alexander's theory is not applicable to the majority of ulcer patients and suggested a theory of multiple etiology. They report that nearly three-fourths (72 percent) of their patients have "typical ulcer personality." Such a personality shows "a strong craving for superiority" and has the following characteristics: drive, versatility, emotional responsiveness, self-reliance, responsibleness, satisfactory sexual adjustment, determination, and a tendency to migrate to larger communities.

   Such personality types for the various psychosomatic disorders, originally suggested by Flanders Dunbar, are not accepted by most authorities.
   (3) Jurgen Ruesch: In a sociopsychological study pointed out that emotions and their influence on gastric secretion and peristalsis are frequently responsible for delayed healing of ulcer, but emphasized that no definite relationship has been established between *initial* ulcer formation and emotions.
       (a) Personality structure shows the ulcer person to be:
           1' Dependent, conforming, overtly counteractive but covertly passive,
           2' Lacking in needs for acquisition, order, and construction, and does not avoid blame,

        3' Most ambivalent about dependence—non-dependence and aggression—nonaggression.

    (b) Socially and culturally:

        1' The social class of the ulcer bearer is primarily lower middle class.

        2' Many were in the process of cultural change.

        3' Acculturation and social mobility are the most important sources of stress for the ulcer bearer.

(4) Current etiological conceptions:

    (a) The role of dependent-independent conflict seems to be accepted by most investigators and is usually related in part to difficulties occurring during the early period of childhood (oral trauma).

    (b) At one time it was thought that persistent, infantile, oral-dependent wishes might lead physiologically to gastric hypersecretion. However, Mirsky's findings suggest that gastric hypersecretion is genetically determined.

(5) It is important to keep in mind psychopathological factors in the overall medical and surgical management of this condition.

4. Irritable bowel syndrome (spastic colon, mucous colitis)

    a. This is a functional bowel disorder characterized by periods of diarrhea, alternating with periods of constipation, abdominal cramps, flatulence, and sometimes by increased mucus in the stool.

    b. These patients are typically obsessive-compulsive in their personality makeup.

    c. Psychological factors must be taken into account in the medical management of this disorder. Effort should be directed at modifying the patients psychological makeup so as to render him less vulnerable to the stresses which are apt to show psychophysiologic reflection in his colon.

5. Ulcerative colitis

    a. Ulcerative colitis is an acute and chronic disease of the mucosa and submucosa of the colon. Bleeding, diarrhea, and abdominal cramps are typical symptoms. Despite much study, the etiology and pathogenesis remains obscure.

b. Emotional disturbances seem to be of some importance at least as contributory factors. This seems particularly true in recurrences.

c. Sometimes the disease seems to develop after prolonged emotional tension.

d. The ulcerative colitis patient has been described as dependent, indecisive, overly conscientious, aggressive, and hostile, although outwardly he may seem self-deprecating. Some have commented on the presence of paranoid tendencies and others have observed neurotic elements with definite compulsive tendencies.

e. Nothing is known of the mechanisms involved in the relationship between psychological stress and the activation of ulcerative colitis.

VI. Psychophysiologic cardiovascular disorders

A. Cardiac neurosis

1. Some authorities still use this term in referring to a patient who has precordial pain, palpitation, dyspnea, and fatigue, but who does not have cardiovascular disease or does not have sufficient cardiovascular pathology to explain his symptoms.

2. In most instances, this is really an anxiety neurosis in which the symptoms are focused chiefly on the heart.

3. Sometimes hyperventilation can produce symptoms of chest pain which simulate heart disease in the mind of the sufferer (see Hyperventilation Syndrome under "Psychophysiologic Respiratory Disorders").

4. Case example: Mr. B., a twenty-five-year-old musician, consulted a psychiatrist complaining of episodes of nervousness, restlessness, palpitation, precordial distress, and a feeling of apprehension ("as if something frightening were going to happen to me"). These episodes began ten months earlier, and he had consulted several physicians during that period of time because he was concerned that he had heart disease. None of the examinations had revealed any evidence of physical disease.

During the first interview, it was learned that his father had been bothered with angina for several years and that two months before the onset of the patient's symptoms, his father had suffered an acute coronary infarction for which he was hospitalized for one month. Shortly after this, the patient developed his first attack of symptoms. Eventually, after several interviews, the patient was able to relate his initial anxiety attack to his father's heart attack and recognize that his continued attacks were really perpetuated by his own guilt from underlying death wishes toward his father that he had repressed for many years.

In this case, note the typical anxiety symptoms which come in attacks and which are focused on the heart. The conflict was relatively superficial and was uncovered fairly rapidly.

B. Essential hypertension
1. This is a systemic reaction in which there is a sustained elevation of blood pressure in the absence of any demonstrable pathology.
2. The etiology is incompletely understood. Most authorities believe that hypertension is caused by an interplay of multiple factors including a psychogenic one. Psychophysiologic studies indicate that the psychogenic component may be closely related to the development of hypertension in some patients and to the production of "hypertensive symptoms" in others.
3. Emotional conflict with the concomitant tension may lead to vasoconstriction and to the subsequent elevation of blood pressure.
4. A continuous struggle against hostile and aggressive impulses is the chief psychogenic factor described by most authorities.
5. Although hypertension occurs in many varieties of personality, it is characteristically found in the person who appears outwardly affable and "easy going," but who suppresses (or represses) hostile and aggressive impulses. When these impulses are frustrated continuously or repeatedly, cardiac symptoms may result. Also he is said to have problems in dependency relationships.
6. Although psychotherapy will lower blood pressure for long periods of time, there are no studies which definitely prove that blood pressure can be permanently lowered by such treatment. The role of emotions is well known (on the clinical course of essential hypertension), but it has not been established that emotional factors are of definite etiological significance.

C. Coronary artery disease
1. Some authorities believe that emotional factors are contributory in angina pectoris and coronary artery disease.

    2. Feelings of failure in the competitive setting or frustrated ambitions have been reported.

D. Vasodepressor syncope

    1. This is fainting due to acute peripheral circulatory inadequacy which is quickly reversible.

    2. It may occur in response to anxiety, pain, shock.

    3. The onset usually occurs while the individual is standing in the erect position and is commonly preceded by anxiety, including sweating, nausea, restlessness, muscle weakness, pallor, and sighing.

    4. Psychophysiologically, it appears that the individual is preparing for action (fight or flight), but neither action occurs. Attacks are more apt to occur if fear is being denied.

E. Migraine

    1. This is a syndrome characterized by recurrent, severe unilateral cephalgia (headache), nausea, vomiting, and scotomata (visual disturbances).

    2. Several factors seem to be of etiological importance, including allergic, hereditary, and psychogenic ones.

    3. The migraine sufferer is said to emphasize the importance of intellectual achievement.

    4. The headache often occurs after periods of stress or hard work rather than during them.

    5. The physiological mechanism has been formulated by H. G. Wolff. In brief, it is a vasoconstriction followed by compensatory vasodilatation in the meningeal arteries, usually of one side only.

    6. Psychopathological aspects

        a. H. G. Wolff sums up the personality characteristics:

            (1) In childhood, the person tended to be sober, polite, and well-mannered, but also showed some contrasting behavior such as stubbornness or inflexibility.

            (2) In adolescence, he was more than usually preoccupied with moralistic and ethical problems.

            (3) In adult life, he was anxious, meticulous, efficient, perfectionistic, exacting, and conservative.

        b. More recent reports in the literature reveal the following:

            (1) Obsessive-compulsive traits are frequently observed. Sensitivity, insecurity, and narcissism are less commonly noted.

            (2) Precipitating factors may be:

        (a) Hostility
        (b) Unresolved dependency
        (c) Nonspecific tensions or frustrations
    (3) Underlying conflicts may be:
        (a) Unexpressed hostility
        (b) Unmet dependency needs
        (c) Multiple or nonspecific conflicts

  c. One gains the impression from recent reports that hostile feelings often trigger the migraine attack but that various conflicts may underlie the hostility. Thus:

$$\text{Conflict (Aroused)} \xrightarrow{\text{leads to}} \text{Hostility (Unexpressed)} \xrightarrow{\text{may produce}} \text{Migraine attack}$$

VII. Psychophysiologic respiratory disorders

A. Various emotions such as hostility, anxiety, fear, or excitement may lead to disturbances in respiration.

B. The respiratory system is involved in one's earliest significant interpersonal relationships and furnishes one of the earliest media of expressing emotional reactions and needs.

C. Hyperventilation syndrome

  1. This is a condition in which the individual is subject to repeated forced respirations, yawning, sensations of air hunger, occasional tetany, chest pain, light-headedness, paresthesias of the hand, feet, and face, and an intense conviction of impending death. Some authorities feel that the hyperventilation syndrome is probably the least recognized anxiety reaction.

  2. It is also known as the effort syndrome, or neurocirculatory asthenia (NCA).

  3. The individual often does not realize that he is over-breathing.

  4. Oftentimes the individual is able to describe the conditions in which the attacks occur. Sometimes they are associated with disturbing dreams.

  5. The hyperventilation syndrome may develop in situations other than emotional stress (e.g., certain febrile illnesses, high altitudes).

  6. Widely divergent emotional states (fear, anxiety, grief, joy, etc.) may lead to the development of hyperventilation. Preoccupation with physical health is usually present in the person who hyperventilates. There is no highly specific

dynamic conflict which leads to this condition, but rather conflicts may be in many different areas.

D. Bronchial asthma

1. This is an allergic disorder with dyspnea and wheezing due to bronchial obstruction resulting from bronchial spasm, bronchial edema, and mucus plugs, in which emotional factors play at least some role.
2. A specific etiology has not been isolated. The most thoroughly investigated one has been hypersensitivity to allergens.
3. Some authorities feel that certain cases of bronchial asthma are primarily psychogenic with repressed hostile feelings being the precipitant of the asthmatic symptomatology.
4. The asthmatic in whom neurotic factors are prominent is thought by some to show unresolved conflict about his dependency on his mother (or mother situation). Sometimes there is fear of abandonment.
5. Thus, the asthmatic attack resembles a suppressed infantile cry (i.e., the attack is actually a cry for help).
6. Pediatricians have commented that asthmatic youngsters cry less readily than nonasthmatic children. The asthmatic wheeze has been likened to the cry of the abandoned child.
7. Psychiatrically oriented medical treatment is the most appropriate approach, thus allowing the asthmatic an opportunity to resolve his dependency problem and deal differently with his underlying hostility.

VIII. **Psychophysiologic genitourinary disorders**

A. Impotence, including premature ejaculation

1. In rare instances impotence is on an organic basis (e.g., multiple sclerosis, drug toxicity). However, in most instances impotence is of psychogenic origin.
2. This condition is also sometimes regarded as a conversion neurosis.
3. Of possible dynamic significance in cases of impotence are the following:
   a. Unresolved oedipal conflict
   b. Fear of female genitalia which are viewed as castrating threats
   c. Latent homosexual strivings
4. Clinically, in cases of impotence occurring in a male who has previously had a long history of sexual adequacy, one will find that the precipitating circumstance often is hostility toward the wife.

   B. Frigidity (including dyspareunia)
1. May be related to fear of pregnancy or fear of being injured during sexual relations.
2. May be related to role identification problems (e.g., envy of masculine role).
   C. Menstrual disorders (including primary amenorrhea and primary dysmenorrhea). These may be related to ambivalence about, or rejection of, the feminine role.
   D. Pseudocyesis (false pregnancy). Is found in women who are strongly desirous of pregnancy and who seem immature and dependent.
   E. Menopausal symptoms
1. Those symptoms which are physiological in origin (hot flashes, excessive perspiration, etc.) are relieved by the administration of hormones.
2. The psychological reaction of the woman to being in the climacterium is discussed under "Involutional Melancholia."

IX. Musculoskeletal disorders
   A. Functional backache: This is often a concern in industrial accidents or compensation cases. (See section on "Compensation Neurosis.")
   B. Tension headache: most commonly related to chronic anxiety.
   C. Rheumatoid arthritis
1. Some observers have reported that the onset or aggravation of rheumatoid arthritis is related to some period of stress. Such individuals are said to be physically active and strongly dependent.
2. Chronic tension and muscular contraction may cause impared circulation and articular changes.
3. Control of hostility is through neuromuscular activity.
4. The physical disability incident to the arthritis may serve as a justification for dependency gratification (this may be true even though the disability is minimal).

X. Psychophysiologic skin disorders
   A. Included here are a number of dermatological reactions such as pruritis, neurodermatitis, hyperhidrosis, angioneurotic-edema.

XI. Emotional reaction to physical illness
   A. Apart from the disorders mentioned (i.e., the recognized psychophysiologic reactions), there are many illnesses in which the patient's psychological reaction may be important.

B. The patient's personality makeup and his emotional needs should be taken into account in the treatment program for any kind of illness.
C. Examples of physical illness which have psychological import:
1. The fourteen-year-old boy who became depressed when he learned that he had diabetes. Beneath the depressive symptoms was the feeling that the diabetes was a punishment for masturbation.
2. The twenty-eight-year-old woman who had been an invalid since age sixteen when she first developed rheumatic heart disease. Although she did have enough heart disease to place some restrictions on her activity, her invalidism (regression) was all out of proportion to the damage to her heart valve. Rehabilitation in this instance was concerned mostly with her emotional reaction to the physical illness.
D. It should be kept in mind that whatever a person's particular illness may be, there usually is a certain amount of accompanying anxiety and this must be recognized and treated.

REFERENCES

Conrad, S. W. "The Psychologic Implications of Overeating." *Psychiat. Quart.* 28(April, 1954):211-224.

Eaton, Merril T., and Peterson, Margaret H. *Psychiatry.* 2nd ed. Flushing, New York: Medical Examination Publishing Company, 1969, chap. VIII.

Freedman, Alfred M.; Kaplan, H. I.; and Sadock, Benjamin J. *Modern Synopsis of Comprehensive Textbook of Psychiatry.* Baltimore: Williams & Wilkins Company, 1972, chap. XXIV.

Kirsner, J. B., and Palmer, W. L. "Ulcerative Colitis." *J.A.M.A.* 155(1954):341.

Kolb, Lawrence C. *Modern Clinical Psychiatry.* 8th ed. Philadelphia: W. B. Saunders Company, 1973, chap. XXV.

Miller, M. L. "Emotional Conflicts in Asthma." *Dis. Nerv. Sys.* 13(October, 1952):298-302

Rowe, C. J., and Lewis, J. S. "Psychodynamic Aspects of Migraine." *Journal-Lancet* 74(1954):95.

Ruesch, Jurgen. *Duodenal Ulcer, A Sociophysiological Study.* Berkeley: University of California Press, 1948.

Sullivan, A. J., and McKell, T. E. *Personality in Peptic Ulcer.* Springfield, Illinois: Charles C. Thomas, Publisher, 1950.

There is something in the character of
every man which cannot be altered:
It is the skeleton of his character.
Trying to change it is like trying to
train sheep to pull a car.

G. C. Lichtenberg: REFLECTIONS, 1799

13

Personality Disorders

Synonyms: character disorders; social deviants

I. **Definition:** These disorders are characterized by deeply ingrained, maladaptive behavioral patterns that are lifelong in duration and often recognizable at adolescence or earlier. At times certain organic disorders of the brain may produce clinical pictures resembling personality disorders. Such conditions are more properly classified under the nonpsychotic organic syndromes.

II. **Personality development**
   A. Personality is the sum total of a person's internal and external patterns of adjustment to life.
   B. Although there may be some variation in his behavior, his adjustment is generally in a state of equilibrium since he has accumulated a repertoire of problem-solving techniques during his period of growth and development.
   C. His personality reflects those coping mechanisms and ego defenses that he uses to maintain his emotional equilibrium.
   D. It also reflects the adjusted compromise that he has made among the pressures from:
      1. Instinctual drives
      2. Reality demands of the environment
      3. Demands of his superego

E. Thus, a person's personality usually reflects the techniques he has for getting along with people in his environment and results from early developmental factors, including the influences of society and culture and childrearing patterns.

III. Characteristics of personality disorder

A. The individual with a personality disorder does not develop symptoms which bother him. In psychoanalytic terminology he has a character neurosis rather than a symptom neurosis.

B. The personality disorder is characterized by it's lifelong nature and the repetitive, maladaptive, often self-defeating behavior (rather than discomfort or symptoms).

C. People with personality disorders are usually anxiety-free except when they are confronted with external stress.

D. Because problems are expressed in a maladaptive form of living rather than symptoms, it is rare for a character-disordered individual to seek help on his own initiative. In general, such people tolerate stress poorly. If they are confronted with minor stresses, they're apt to become anxious; or if confronted with moderate stresses may develop transient psychotic reactions.

E. It should be remembered that many of the difficulties people have adjusting to the world may be due to social stress or disarrangement rather than disordered character (e.g., chapter on "Transient Situational Disturbances").

IV. Etiological factors: Included as possible causal factors are:

A. Constitutional predisposition

B. Childhood experiences which have fostered deviant behavior

  1. When acting-out behavior is rewarded (such as temper tantrums or hostile-aggressive behavior); or, when overly conforming behavior is encouraged and creativity is discouraged.

  2. Circumstances in which normal behavior is not allowed to develop, as for example, the rigid, unreasonable parent who adamantly refuses to accept any reason for nonconformity.

C. Identification with parents or other authority figures who have similar deviancies.

V. Types of personality disorders

A. Included under this classification are:

  1. Personality disorders (301)

  2. Sexual deviations (302)

3. Alcoholism (303)
4. Drug dependence (304)

B. This chapter will describe all of the personality disorders listed under "1" above with the exception of Antisocial Personality which will be discussed in a separate chapter.

VI. Personality disorders (301)

✱A. Paranoid personality

1. Definition: People with this personality type show hypersensitivity, rigidity, unwarranted suspicion, jealousy, envy, excessive self-importance, and a tendency to blame others and ascribe evil motives to them. They show a conspicuous tendency to overuse the mechanism of projection.

2. Etiology:
   a. See Etiological Factors above
   b. Some think that the paranoid personalities often had opposite sex parents who were domineering, overprotective, and ambivalent and same sex parents who were submissive, passive, and relatively unavailable to the child "as an object for identification." (Freeman et al.)

3. Case example: J. H., a thirty-eight-year-old married man, was referred to the court psychiatric consultant for evaluation after he had pleaded guilty to a charge of assault growing out of a complaint filed by his wife whom he had beaten up one evening in a bar. He admitted to one previous court appearance for leaving the scene of an accident and also admitted to being jailed overnight once for drunkenness. On interview, he admitted to having beaten his wife once previously, but tended to minimize this by saying that he only slapped her with his open hand. He admitted to arguing with his wife but tended to minimize it by saying it was not too much different than most married couples. His wife reported that he carried a chip on his shoulder most of the time and felt that people owed him something. She indicated that he was "very suspicious" of her friends and that he would not talk with them. He constantly suspected that his wife was unfaithful and was unable to place trust and confidence in physicians even though by neglecting to do so, he had impaired his health. His Minnesota Multiphasic Personality Inventory profile was consistent with a diagnosis of paranoid personality. He seemed to be the sort of person who could keep his paranoid feelings under

good control as long as he did not drink. Whenever he did drink, his suspicions and projections became more prominent and he acted on them.

*B. Cyclothymic personality (affective personality):
  1. Definition: People in this group show recurring and alternating periods of depression and elation. The periods of elation may be characterized by ambition, warmth, enthusiasm, optimism and high energy, or if severe, may approach grandiosity. The periods of depression may be marked by worry, pessimism, low energy, and a sense of futility, or they may become immobilizing.
  2. Cyclothymic personality is sometimes described as miniature manic-depressive illness. Differentiation from manic-depressive illness is largely a matter of degree.
  3. Case example: P. D., a thirty-year-old married man was referred for psychiatric evaluation by his attorney to whom he had gone to confer about a rather grandiose scheme to make money by purchasing several small companies. He actually had no money and a very bad credit rating because of previous financial reverses. When he presented himself at the psychiatrist's office he immediately greeted the receptionist by her first name (although he had never met her before) and then visited brightly with several people in the reception room in a very friendly, breezy manner. When interviewed by the psychiatrist, he was exuberant, glib, and loquacious. At the end of the hour, he admitted he felt "a bit high" and said that most of the time he was an extrovertive, verbal, outgoing, and exuberant person. However, he did admit that he had brief periods when he slowed down and felt gloomy. He also gave a history of a frank depressive episode two years earlier for which he had received electroshock therapy.

*C. Schizoid personality
  1. Definition: People with this type of personality manifest shyness, oversensitivity, seclusiveness, avoidance of close or competitive relationships, and often eccentricity. Autistic thinking and daydreaming are common, and they are often unable to express hostile and aggressive feelings.
  2. The point at which a schizoid personality becomes schizophrenic is often times arbitrary.
  3. Case example: C. N., a twenty-five-year-old single girl, was referred to the court psychiatric consultant for evaluation

after she had been arrested in the lobby of a downtown hotel for drunkenness. Aside from her drunken state, there was no other behavioral disturbance that had brought her to the attention of the authorities. She had never been arrested previously. On examination, she was very quiet and verbalized little or nothing. Most of the information obtained from her was through a question-and-answer approach. She responded to direct questions, but volunteered very little about herself. She had a somewhat disheveled appearance and wore an unusual amount of cheap jewelry. Although she was a college graduate, she was working as a cocktail waitress in one of the local country clubs. She readily admitted to having a drinking problem and estimated that about twice a month she drank to the point that she blacked out. Most of her drinking was done while she was alone, although some of it was done in the company of some of the other waitresses. She did not seem to be very introspective or reflective. When asked to give her opinion of herself, she replied by saying that she never thought much about herself. She admitted to being very passive and said that she felt easily led. She admitted to feelings of inferiority and did not look ahead as to what she might do in the future. The probation officer who had investigated her reported that she was a very shy, withdrawn person, sadly lacking in self-confidence.

D. Explosive personality (epileptoid personality disorder)
1. Definition: People with this disorder have uncontrollable gross outbursts of rage or of verbal or physical aggressiveness. Such outbursts are in contrast to the person's usual behavior and he may regret and repent them afterwards. Such people are generally excitable, aggressive, and over-responsive to environmental pressure.
2. In the absence of stress, such persons may seem pleasant and well adjusted. However, when confronted with seemingly insignificant events, they become enraged.
3. Case example: A twenty-two-year-old married man was referred to the court psychiatric consultant for evaluation after he had pleaded guilty to a charge of simple assault, growing out of an incident in which he was verbally and physically abusive to his wife. He was on probation at the time of the offense for a similar disorderly conduct offense committed nine months earlier.

At the interview he was cooperative and pleasant but did not spontaneously volunteer much about himself. He was quiet, nonverbal, and not at all reflective. Concerning his difficulty, he said, "basically it's temper" which had been an issue in his marriage for the preceding three years. He said that the difficulty was that his temper began during the time that he was in the service for two years following his eighteenth birthday. "It just seemed to come on by itself." It had its onset shortly before he was sent overseas to Vietnam where he served as an infantry rifleman and was wounded.

The kind of anger with the subsequent physical and verbal abuse of his wife occurred about every six months. At such times he usually would awaken angry and as a consequence, would overreact throughout the entire day.

Mental status evaluation revealed him to be free of anxiety and depression. He didn't think that there was anything wrong with his mind and he denied delusions, hallucinations, and other types of perceptual distortions. He denied any thinking disturbance. He thought that it was sometimes hard for him to trust others.

It was the consultant's opinion that this man had an explosive personality. Since the outbursts seemed to develop in relationships chiefly with his wife, it was suggested that they both be referred for marriage counseling if the wife planned to remain in the marriage.

E. Obsessive-compulsive personality
1. Definition: People with this personality type show excessive concern with conformity and adherence to standards of conscience. Thus, such individuals are rigid, overinhibitive, overconscientious, overdutiful, and unable to relax easily. This personality type may lead into obsessive-compulsive neurosis.
2. Etiology
   a. The person who possesses such traits is referred to as an *anancastic personality* or anal character (such an individual needs to feel in control of himself and his environment).
   b. According to psychoanalytic theory, such anal qualities develop in the infant during the period of toilet training (the anal phase of infantile sexuality).
   c. According to learning theory, obsessions are conditioned stimulus responses to anxiety and compulsions are behavioral patterns which reduce the anxiety.

3. Case example: A fifty-two-year-old financial officer of a large corporation consulted a psychiatrist because of his conflict in his relationships with his wife and his business associates. At the first interview he stated that he was a very conscientious, inflexible, punctual, conforming man who had technically performed his financial services to the corporation flawlessly. However, the very traits which made his financial calculations so accurate also rendered him relatively inflexible in dealing with human beings. For example, he was very critical of his boss and his fellow workers for being late to work or for any infractions of company policy or rules. With his wife, he was critical of her in matters of neatness, punctuality, and her housework.

He planned to continue in treatment to help himself become more flexible.

F. Hysterical personality (histrionic personality disorder):
   1. Definition: People with this personality type show excitability, emotional instability, overreactivity and self-dramatization. The self-dramatization is always attention-seeking and often seductive. Such people are often immature, self-centered, usually dependent, and often have an overly optimistic, overly nice attitude toward life.
   2. See section on Psychopathology under Hysterical Neurosis.
   3. From the psychoanalytic viewpoint, the hysterical personality is fixated at the oral level of sexual development.
   4. Case examples:
      a. Wilkins Micawber, the impecunious comic character in *David Copperfield* by Charles Dickens, seems to be a hysterical type of character. Although spending himself into Debtor's Prison and eking out a shabby existence, he is "always waiting for something to turn up."
      ✱b. Scarlet O'Hara, the heroine of Margaret Mitchell's; *Gone With The Wind,* seems to be a hysterical character. At the end of the novel, after she is rejected by Rhett Butler, she can't think of letting him go and thinks, "I won't think of it now—I'll go home to Tara tomorrow—I'll think of it all tomorrow at Tara. I can stand it then. Tomorrow, I'll think of some way to get him back. After all, tomorrow is another day."

G. Asthenic personality
   1. Definition: People with this type of personality show easy fatigability, lasitude, low energy level, lack of enthusiasm, marked incapacity for enjoyment (anhedonia), lack of will

(abulia), and oversensitivity to physical and emotional stress. Such individuals may develop neurasthenic neurosis.

2. Case example: A fifty-five-year-old Roman Catholic Nun sought psychiatric consultation because of tiredness, exhaustion, easy fatigability, and depression. A report from her superior indicated that she had always been a conscientious and efficient teacher and she had had no problems in her relationships with the other nuns, the parents, the children, or authority.

   She gave a history of having fatigued easily and being possessed of a very low energy level all of her life. As she got older, she required more and more rest and sleep to perform the same tasks that she had earlier in life. For example, after the age of forty-eight she would usually become extremely fatigued about March of each academic year and go to bed as soon as she ate an early supper and remain in bed for at least twelve hours. She sought assistance from the psychiatrist in being excused from any education activities during the summer months because she required that period to restore her energy level to a point where she could again resume classroom teaching in the fall.

H. Passive-aggressive personality
   1. Definition: People with this type of personality show both passivity and aggressivity. The aggressiveness may be expressed in such passive ways as obstructionism, pouting, procrastination, intentional inefficiency, or stubbornness. Such behavior usually reflects hostility which the individual feels he dare not express openly. Often the behavior is an expression of his resentment at his inability to find gratification in a relationship with an individual or institution upon which he is overdependent.
   2. Subtypes
      a. Passive-dependent type: Such a person is clinging, indecisive, and helpless. Such behavior may be a disguised means of controlling or manipulating others.
      b. Passive-aggressive type: Hostile and destructive wishes are expressed through such covert ways as procrastination, obstructionism, and stubbornness.
   3. Case example: F. S., a thirty-four-year-old married man, was referred to the court psychiatric consultant for evaluation after he had pleaded guilty to a charge of assault and battery and drunkenness upon a complaint filed by his

wife, who reported that he came home drunk and threatened her with a knife. He had one previous arrest as a juvenile for malicious destruction of property and two prior arrests as an adult, one for drunkenness and the other for drunken driving. Upon interview, he blamed his drinking on his family troubles. He felt there had been lots of pressures within his marriage for the preceding three or four years and particularly implicated his father-in-law as playing a prominent role in the conflict between him and his wife. He was critical of his wife and said that she was shiftless and dominated by her mother, although faithful. He felt that he was unable to communicate with either his father-in-law or his wife because they were both illiterate. Although he admitted that most of his complaints about his wife were minor ones, he felt they all added up to incompatibility in his marriage. He felt that his wife constantly aggravated him by her behavior and that this led to numerous arguments and difficulties. When not drinking, he was passive and not at all aggressive in his behavior toward his wife. He had consulted numerous physicians for various physical problems, including hypoglycemia. He had been unemployed for the preceding year. There was no history of aggressive behavior toward other people nor had he ever been involved in altercations with men.

I. Inadequate personality
   1. Definition: People with this type of personality show ineffectual responses to emotional, social, intellectual, and physical demands. They manifest inadaptability, ineptness, poor judgment, social instability, and lack of physical and emotional stamina.
   2. Case example: J. S., a thirty-three-year-old single woman, was referred to the court psychiatric consultant for evaluation after she had pleaded guilty to a charge of disorderly conduct growing out of an incident in which she was picked up on suspicion of having dropped matches in a mailbox, and after having behaved suspiciously in the doorways of business establishments in the same area. She had no record of previous arrests. On interview, she appeared somewhat disheveled. Her hair was combed back straight and she wore rather thick glasses. Nystagmoid movements of the eyes were noted and she spoke in a rather high-pitched voice. According to the presentence study, she had changed her story on two or three occasions, at first admit-

ting that she had thrown the matches into the mailbox when investigated by the postal authorities and later changing her story about this. She seemed withdrawn and emotionally disturbed. Her IQ evaluations obtained from school records indicated that her IQ ranged from 91 to 100. Actually, her behavior and school achievement would suggest that her IQ level was lower. She had few friends and was described as a "loner." She had never been able to hold a regular job but had worked for short periods of time at one of the local Goodwill Industries. She had been described by friends as goodhearted but childish. Others had noted that she was not too well mannered and was difficult to handle. She had almost no interests. Mostly she cared for her own apartment and visited a disabled lady friend who lived several blocks away. At the time of arrest, she was employed in a local community workshop. During the interview, she gave the impression of being dull, simple, and strange. There was no evidence during the interview nor on psychological testing that she was psychotic.

J. Antisocial personality (see next chapter)

VII. Treatment

A. Therapy of these "basic" personality types is very difficult because they usually lack any fundamental motivation for change.

B. When they do seek treatment, it is often likely to be:
1. Because of anxiety developing secondarily to the social repercussions of their behavior.
2. At the insistence of another person (a parent, spouse, or employer).
3. Because of the slowly developing awareness of an unsatisfactory life-style.

C. The positive rewards from their behavior over balances the socially incurred ill-feeling that may result.

D. In individual therapy, the therapist may focus on the individual's maladaptive behavior rather than on a discussion of his inner life.

E. Oftentimes such persons need a different model with whom to identify and from whom to obtain reliable feedback about the nature of their emotional impact on others. In general, the therapist must remain flexible and be prepared to take an active role in the treatment process if necessary.

F. Group therapy has been of some value.

REFERENCES

American Psychiatric Association. *Diagnostic and Statistical Manual of Mental Disorders*. 2nd ed. Washington, D.C., 1968. Seventh Printing, July 1974.

Eaton, M. T., Jr., and Peterson, M. H. *Psychiatry*. 2nd ed. Flushing, New York: Medical Examination Publishing Company, 1969, chap. VII.

Freedman, A. M.; Kaplan, H. I.; and Sadock, B. J. *Modern Synopsis of Comprehensive Textbook of Psychiatry*. Baltimore: Williams & Wilkins, 1972, chap. XX.

Kolb, Lawrence C. *Modern Clinical Psychiatry*. 8th ed. Philadelphia: W. B. Saunders Company, 1973, chap. XXVI.

Solomon, P. D., and Patch, V. D. *Handbook of Psychiatry*. 2nd ed. Los Altos, California: Lang Medical Publication, 1971, chap. XVII.

When a rogue kisses you,
Count your teeth.

Hebrew Proverb

Antisocial Personality

Synonyms: sociopathic personality disturbance; psychopathic personality, sociopath; psychopath, semantic disorder; moral imbecile

I. **Definition:** A person who is basically unsocialized and whose behavior patterns bring him into repeated conflict with society. He manifests his conflict by "acting out" behavior toward his environment. His behavior is chiefly antisocial, asocial, and amoral in character.

II. **Occurrence**
   A. The exact incidence is not known partly because of the lack of agreement among authorities as to what kind of personality disturbance should be classified as antisocial.
   B. Public mental hospitals show low admission rates for antisocial personalities. However, this probably does not reflect the actual incidence of the disorder, since many antisocial personalities are excluded from hospitalization or are sentenced to jails or prisons for their offenses against society. Most hospitals try to exclude antisocial persons from admission because they are not really equipped to deal with them.
   C. Most people with antisocial personality are found in the lower socioeconomic groups, coming largely from backgrounds of rejection, deprivation, neglect, and abuse.

D. The sex incidence is preponderantly male (estimates are that five to ten times as many males receive this diagnosis).

III. Symptoms

A. The onset of antisocial behavior is often before the age of fifteen.

B. Traits found in childhood
   1. Typically, the child is dominated by primitive drives and lacks socialization of his behavior.
   2. He shows emotional immaturity and impulsivity.
   3. Frequently he is destructive, deceitful, obstinate, quarrelsome, and defiant.
   4. He may show temper tantrums or outbursts of rage.
   5. Delinquent behavior, such as theft, truancy, running away, pathological lying, and incorrigibility are common.
   6. Enuresis is common.

C. Traits found in adolescence
   1. Rebelliousness against parental or other forms of authority.
   2. Resistance to accepting the value system of his family.
   3. He may show conflict with school authorities and show poor academic performance.
   4. As he approaches adulthood, all of these traits may become exaggerated because of the increased responsibility he has to cope with as well as the weakening of the restraining forces of the family ties.

D. Traits found in adult life
   1. Emotional immaturity and impulsivity. Like a child he is unwilling to subordinate his own desires to the wishes of the others and he follows the desires of the moment.
   2. Antisocial, asocial, or amoral behavior. Because his defective conscience allows him to gratify his impulses, he does not have to regard moral, ethical, or social limitations on his actions. He frequently has a police record.
   3. Egocentricity and selfishness. He is so self-centered that he is incapable of object love. Thus, he has difficulty in relating to others and for this reason lacks any lasting close personal relationships. Hence, he poses difficulty in psychiatric treatment.
   4. Poor judgment. Lack of judgment or defective judgment is very characteristic of the antisocial person.
   5. Unreliability and undependability. He has no sense of responsibility, although at first glance he often appears reliable. He disregards the truth; he often lies about the past

and makes unkept promises for the future. (In dealing with the antisocial person, one should base predictions about future behavior on his past performances rather than on his well-intentioned promises.)

6. Lack of appreciation for the consequences of his actions. He is unwilling to accept the blame for any of his misfortunes.

7. Inability to tolerate frustration. He follows the pleasure principle and is uninfluenced by the reality principle.

8. Inability to postpone immediate gratification. This is related to his immaturity, egocentricity, and impulsivity (he expects immediate gratification—he wants what he wants when he wants it).

9. Conflict with, or defiance of, authority. This is related to his earlier interpersonal relationships with parents, parent surrogates, or other authority figures.

10. Inability to profit from experience. He never learns from his mistakes and seems uninfluenced by reason or punishment. (Punishment seems to be no deterrent at all.)

11. He is relatively free of anxiety, remorse, or guilt.

12. Abuse of alcohol and drugs. He often abuses alcohol and may take drugs of various kinds for their pleasurable effects.

13. Projections of his own shortcomings onto the world. He seeks the explanation for his difficulty in the environment rather than within himself and tends to blame everyone or everything but himself.

14. Poor occupational adjustment. His job performance, attendance, and efficiency are often erratic or poor. He finds routine boring and sometimes intolerable.

15. An inner conviction that he is immune to the usual social customs and laws. This is seen repeatedly in the antisocial person, particularly the one who comes in conflict with the law. Although he seems to have an intellectual awareness that people are expected to behave in a certain way or to conform to certain standards, he appears to regard himself as an exception to these standards.

E. The less aggressive antisocial person is often outwardly appealing.

F. The pattern of behavioral disturbance is often monotonous and repetitious. He shows the same poor judgment repeatedly. (This is seen classically in those who commit crimes. The crime is usually similar—for example, a check forger usually does not commit aggressive types of crimes, but only writes "rubber checks.")

G. Though the behavior is commonly socially destructive or hostile, some sociopaths seem to act as if they were being self-destructive or were seeking punishment.

H. Antisocial behavior begins in late childhood or early adolescence, tends to become more severe in early adult life, and may diminish in late middle life (those who level off in later years in the past were referred to as "burned out psychopaths").

IV. Etiology

A. The causes of antisocial personality are not really known.

B. Earlier reports stressed the "constitutional" aspects of the disorder. Such emphasis grew out of the observations of those who noted the beginning of difficulty with parents in early years and a continuing difficulty in interpersonal relationships throughout life. Since the course seemed so inexorable, constitutionality was invoked as the chief etiological factor.

C. Some cases of antisocial behavior have been precipitated by brain damage, as for example, severe head trauma or encephalitis. Although the behavior here may be classified as antisocial, technically such individuals are not usually considered to be antisocial personalities, but rather are more properly considered as having organic brain syndromes.

D. Psychological and social factors are believed to be chiefly responsible for the development of the antisocial personality disturbance.

   1. Social factors
      a. The antisocial personality comes largely from the lower socioeconomic groups. There is a high rate of delinquency in the slum areas of larger urban communities.
      b. Living according to the pleasure principle without regard for the reality principle is in part determined by social factors (as well as parental relationships).
      c. The families and environment from which antisocial persons come show high rates of broken homes, alcoholism, antisocial behavior.
   2. Psychological factors
      a. Early experiences, especially in relationships with parents or parent substitutes are regarded as most significant.

    b. The hallmark of the antisocial personality is the relative absence of a socialized superego.

    c. The families and environment from which antisocial persons come show high rates of broken homes, al-immediate satisfactions by himself and attempting to control and manipulate others.

V. Psychopathology

  A. The essential defect in the antisocial personality involves his character structure (hence this disturbance is sometimes called a character disorder or character neurosis).

  B. Like the infant, the antisocial personality gives direct expression to his impulses. He is seemingly incapable of adapting his inner urges to the demands of society and is unable to postpone immediate gratification of his desires.

  C. He defies, or comes in conflict with, authority and lacks sensitivity for other people's feelings.

  D. Since he is dominated by his nonsocialized drives, he has difficulty in his interpersonal relationships with other people. Although intellectually he recognizes that his acts are illegal or unethical, he seems uninfluenced by such knowledge.

  E. He might be considered emotionally deficient. He is egocentric, selfish, makes excessive demands, and is unable to view his own behavior objectively. He is usually free of anxiety, remorse, or guilt.

  F. From the foregoing, it becomes apparent that the antisocial person has a poorly developed conscience ("defective superego").

    1. Conscience is largely dependent upon relationships with parents or parent substitutes. Usually one's value system is something one develops through his relationships with parents (largely by identification) and is based on affection and trust.

    2. In the antisocial person, the identification process is faulty. Either he is unable to evolve a value system through the normal process of identification or he shows the pathological types of identification.

      a. Hostile identification: Internalization of undesirable personality traits of parents or authority figures, or

      b. Identification with the aggressor: Internalization of the characteristics of a frustrated or feared parent or parent substitute.

3. In the antisocial person, we often find that there is a history of difficulty with parents or authority figures from the earliest years.
4. This seems related to parental attitudes which are commonly unreasonable, neglectful, cruel, hypocritical, or inconsistent (i.e., vacillating or unpredictable). A child has difficulty attaching himself to either parent as an example to follow or as a source of security (because there has been a lack of mutual affection, tenderness, or trust).
5. Because of this detachment from parents and parent-figures, his behavior develops no sense of direction (that is, he is uninfluenced by any concepts of right and wrong).
6. In a sense, some authorities feel that his willful, unsocialized behavior is a seeking for attention, affection, and acceptance.

VI. **Case report:** Bob, the eighteen-year-old son of well-to-do parents, was brought to the hospital for psychiatric examination upon the order of a judge. One night four weeks earlier the patient in the company of three other boys entered a cemetery, tipped over several gravestones, and mutilated a monument.

When Bob first entered grade school, he had some minor difficulties. He performed below his intellectual capacity and frequently did things that the other children considered "daring," such as letting the air out of automobile tires. At age nine, he began to smoke, not just experimentally like some of the other boys, but often and somewhat defiantly.

He first came into difficulty with the law at the age of eleven when he stole two cigarette lighters and a wristwatch from a jewelry store. Following this, he was sent to a military boarding school upon the advice of the judge and the family physician. Two months after he entered the new school, he broke into the school store, stole candy and cigarettes and ran away to a nearby city. He was found two days later in a hotel room by himself. He was returned to his parental home and finished the remainder of the school year at the local school. At the age of thirteen, he and two other boys stole a large amount of gasoline from a nearby storage plant. This was used in a "jalopy" purchased for the patient by his father. At first he denied the theft, but when confronted with irrefutable proof, he admitted his guilt; however, he was unable to give any reason for wanting the gasoline. From the age of thirteen until age seventeen, he was frequently involved in minor delinquencies but always escaped punishment because of his family's respected position in the community and because his father always made restitution. At the age of seventeen, he began drinking beer and shortly was getting "high" quite regularly.

Bob was the older of two brothers but was really reared as an only child since his brother died in infancy when Bob was four. After this, the parents overindulged him. At the age of five, he fell from a horse following which he had a few convulsions. He was examined at a well-known clinic and placed on anticonvulsants and a ketogenic diet. After a few weeks of this treatment, he quit taking the medications, buried the special dietary foods and stole bread to eat. He says he has never been really close to anyone and has never felt toward his parents as other youngsters do. Although the parents verbally disapproved of his behavior, they encouraged it in subtle ways; for example, increasing his already overly generous allowance after he was caught stealing from a hardware store.

At no time has he ever shown any guilt for his delinquent and antisocial behavior, and he always seems free of anxiety.

This case illustrates some of the typical aspects of the antisocial person.

VII. Impulse neurosis (impulse-ridden state)

A. Not all antisocial behavior is identified with persons diagnosed antisocial personalities, any more than all episodes of intoxification are found exclusively in alcohol addicts.

B. Excluded from the Antisocial Personality disorders are a group called neurotic characters, or acting-out neurotics, whose disturbance is characterized by the irresistible, repetitious expression of a *single*, pleasurable impulse.

C. It may be the expression of any type of impulse. Some have sexual significance, such as exhibitionism. There are others:
   1. Kleptomania, Neurotic stealing
   2. Pyromania, Neurotic fire-setting

D. The specific symptom has a symbolic significance and is related to the patient's life history.

E. In these disorders, the superego is usually well developed and is only defective to the extent that it permits acting out one type of antisocial behavior.

VIII. Prognosis

A. In general, the prognosis for antisocial personality is not good. However, periods of remission and improvement apparently do occur in some individuals with this reaction.

B. Some antisocial persons level off in later life as previously mentioned.

    C. Impulse neurotics often respond to psychotherapy so that the prognosis is more hopeful.

IX. Treatment

    A. Since the antisocial person does not think of himself as ill, he rarely, if ever, seeks treatment voluntarily.

    B. Treatment is extremely difficult and generally has been unsuccessful.

    C. Those methods of management which have been based chiefly on punishment and reasoning usually have failed.

    D. Treatment is directed at attempting to help the individual develop internal controls. The therapist or counselor who can develop a warm, authoritative, father-figure image can often have positive influence on such persons, particularly if his therapeutic position is heavily ladened with patience and tolerance.

    E. Some authorities believe that therapy should be directed at developing a functioning conscience by having the therapist serve as a model for the patient. This treatment obviously is very difficult but apparently has met with limited success.

    F. Group therapy in selected settings seems to have been of some help in developing social consciences in these people.

    G. Some authorities have suggested establishing special hospitals to evaluate and treat the antisocial person. This position has some merit since most of the hospitals admitting psychiatric patients at the present time are not structured to deal with such people. Imprisonment usually does not help.

    H. Ordinarily, the psychiatrist should avoid prescribing drugs for the antisocial personality.

REFERENCES

Bosselman, B. C. *Neurosis and Psychosis.* 3rd ed. Springfield, Illinois: Charles C. Thomas, 1964, chap. VI and VII.

Cleckley, H. *The Mask of Sanity.* 4th ed. St Louis: C. V. Mosby Company, 1964.

Eaton, M. T., Jr., and Peterson, M. H. *Psychiatry.* 2nd ed. Flushing, New York: Medical Examination Publishing Company, 1969, chap. XIV.

Freedman, A. M.; Kaplan, H. I.; and Sadock, B. J. *Modern Synopsis of Comprehensive Textbook of Psychiatry.* Baltimore: Williams & Wilkins, 1972, chap. XX.

Hirschfeld, A. H. and Behan, Robert C. "The Accident Process—An Overview." *Journal of Rehabilitation,* January-February 1967.

Kolb, L. C. *Modern Clinical Psychiatry.* 8th ed. Philadelphia: W. B. Saunders Company, 1973, chap. XVI.

Sexual Deviations

Synonyms: sexual perversion; paraphilia

I. Definition: Any aberrant sexual behavior which is predominantly preferred to, or takes the place of, normal heterosexual behavior.

II. Concepts of sexual deviancy
    A. Sexual deviations have been practiced throughout history and have been present among all races.
    B. Some deviant acts may be considered to be within the normal range of sexual expression if indulged in only sporatically or as foreplay preceding normal coitus.
    C. Sexual deviancy includes any sexual behavior which is at variance with more or less culturally accepted norms.
    D. Either the quality of the sexual drives or the object of the sexual drives is abnormal.
    E. Like the neuroses there is internal conflict, but like the personality disorders there is character defect—thus allowing the individual to "act out" his conflict through sexual deviancy rather than developing anxiety or other neurotic symptoms.
    F. Those who are heterosexually oriented under normal conditions but who, because they are segregated from the opposite sex for long periods of time, casually seek sexual gratification through the various perversions, are not sexual deviates in the

119

strict sense of the definition (e.g., prisoners). Such people are sometimes referred to as incidental deviates.

G. Outwardly, sexual deviants seem normal.

H. Deviant sexual acts usually have an impulsive and compulsive aspect.

III. Etiology

A. There are theories to explain sexual deviation, but the proven facts concerning etiology are quite scanty.

B. At one time hormone imbalance had been thought by a few authorities to play some role in sexual deviation. However, most laboratory studies do not substantiate such theories.

C. Constitutional factors are usually not considered to be of any major etiological significance in the sexual deviations. Even among those who feel constitution may play some role, it is believed that early experiences are important as well.

D. Some feel that sociocultural factors play a role in the development of homosexuality or prohibitions against it.

E. Sexual deviation is almost universally regarded as psychogenic in origin.

1. Tendencies towards deviancy are latently present in everyone. The forces most commonly hypothesized as making these tendencies overt are:

   a. Castration anxiety.

   b. Oedipal conflicts.

   c. Certain abnormalities of family interaction during the deviant's childhood years.

2. Most authorities consider the roots of origin to be in the early stages of psychosexual development, essentially within the infantile sexual forces.

3. When there is fixation at, or regression back to, these early stages, together with a fixating experience, sexual deviancy results.

   a. According to Freudian theory, the regression or fixation was in the pregential level or "polymorphus perverse" stage. Pleasure was obtained from nongenital, autoerotic activities. Thus, certain sexual behavior common at earlier stages may persist (or reappear later). For example, if the looking and exhibiting common in the small child persists into adult life, they are regarded as sexual deviations (voyeurism and exhibitionism).

4. A boy with an aggressive, dominating mother and a passive, submissive father may have difficulty in his role identification.

    5. Similarly, a young girl with a mother who has been dissatisfied with her role as wife and mother may have difficulty in making a good adult, feminine identification.

  F. According to psychoanalytic theory, these deviations are derived primarily from infantile sexuality. Of central importance in understanding the deviant behavior is the presence of underlying castration anxiety and the unresolved oedipal situation. The deviation is seen as an acted-out denial of castration anxiety. Freud believed that the sexual deviations were "the negative of neurosis" and that the deviant was giving direct and exaggerated expression of instincts rather than repressing them and expressing them symbolically as was done by the neurotic.

  G. The deviant is narcissistic and the impulse he acts out is pleasurable (ego-syntonic).

IV. Prognosis: In most cases of sexual deviancy, the prognosis is poor since there is little motivation for change in behavior.

V. Varieties of sexual deviations
  A. Homosexuality*
  B. Fetishism
  C. Pedophilia
  D. Transvestitism
  E. Transsexualism
  F. Exhibitionism
  G. Voyeurism
  H. Sadism
  I. Masochism
  J. Other sexual deviation

VI. Homosexuality (Sexual orientation disturbance)
  A. Definition: Sexual attraction or desire for sexual contact with a person of the same sex. The individual is psychologically of one sex and physically of the opposite sex. Homosexual behavior in females is also called *lesbianism*.
  B. Occurrence
    1. It is the most common of sexual deviations.

---

*In December, 1973 the Board of Trustees of the American Psychiatric Association substituted for homosexuality a new definition and category: *Sexual Orientation Disturbance*. This category is for individuals whose sexual interests are directed primarily toward people of the same sex and who are either disturbed by, in conflict with, or wish to change their sexual orientation. This diagnostic category is distinguished from homosexuality, which by itself, does not necessarily constitute a psychiatric disorder. This decision was upheld by a substantial majority in a referendum of the voting members of the association in May, 1974.

2. According to Kinsey's survey, about 4 percent of caucasian males consider themselves homosexuals.
3. It is found in all socioeconomic classes.
4. Homosexuals tend to congregate largely in urban areas where they often make contacts ("pickups") at gay bars, or by "cruising" on the public streets. Male homosexuals also make contacts in steam baths.

C. Types of homosexual behavior
1. Some openly live the homosexual life. Others are more discreet and live in the heterosexual world.
2. There are two major groupings of male homosexuals:
   a. Those males who are exclusively homosexual in their behavior and orientation.
   b. A second group in whom homosexuality is less prominent. Men in this latter group live in the heterosexual world and by-and-large lead heterosexual lives (are married and have families). They carry out their homosexual lives in secret and only relatively infrequently (such men are known in the gay world as "closet queens").
3. Certain occupations have an overrepresentation of homosexual persons. In males there is an overrepresentation in acting, interior decorating, dancing, and hairdressing. In females there is an overrepresentation in trucking, engineering, and mechanical types of work.

D. Etiology
1. See Etiology under Sexual Deviations at the beginning of the chapter.
2. Constitutional factors
   a. Heterosexual and homosexual components are found in the libidinal drives of everyone. Our sexual behavior is related to our identification and also our ability to sublimate certain drives.
   b. A surfacing of homosexual drives has been attributed by some to genetic or biologic factors.
3. Psychoanalytic theory
   a. According to this theory, homosexuality is based on the underlying castration anxiety and unresolved oedipal situations.
   b. The male homosexual has identified with his mother.
   c. The female homosexual has identified with her father.
4. Environmental theories
   a. Some authorities believe that homosexual men have overly close, overly intimate, possessive, dominating,

overprotective and "demasculinizing" mothers, and detached, unaffectionate, hostile fathers who treat their sons in a humiliating way.
   b. Similarly, homosexual females are said to have submissive fathers who were distant to their daughters, and mothers who were hostile, competitive, and defeminizing and who favored sons.
   c. Seduction in early life by a homosexual may play a significant etiological role in certain cases.
5. Cultural theories
   a. Homosexuality has been found in both past and present cultures. It has been viewed by some as a normal variant of our biological behavior. However, there are cultures in which homosexuality is unknown.
   b. Subcultures in which there is an undue restriction on any show of heterosexual interest (such as prohibition of dating, dancing, etc.) may lead to the belief that homosexual behavior is less forbidden than heterosexual behavior.
   c. Homosexuality may occur transiently. As for example, in adolescents as an expression of curiosity or experimentation, or in certain circumstances where heterosexual contacts are unavailable, as for example, prison.
E. Clinical types
   1. Latent homosexuality: The homosexual desires are largely unconscious, unrecognized, and sublimated. Latency varies inversely with the strength of repression.
   2. Overt homosexuality: Homosexuality which is recognized consciously.
      a. Most homosexuals are normal in appearance.
      b. Some show some of the outward behavioral characteristics of the opposite sex. For example, some male homosexuals are effeminate in appearance and manner and some homosexual women seem aggressive and masculine.
F. Treatment
   1. Of the basic underlying homosexuality
      a. Intensive psychotherapy, or psychoanalysis has been reported as having favorable results in a significant number who sought treatment and wanted change.
      b. Behavior modification treatment: Negative conditioning in which homoerotic pictures have been shown and then accompanied by injection of apomorphone (to

produce vomiting), or painful electrical stimuli has been tried as an aversion technique. Some favorable results have been reported.
c. Drug therapy
   (1) Tranquilizers or antidepressants for the existence of coincidental anxiety or depression.
   (2) Male hormones in male homosexuality seem contraindicated since they only increase the sexual drive without changing the aim.
d. Group therapy has been said to have beneficial results.
2. Of incidental neurotic symptoms or personality problems: in general follows the same rules as apply for heterosexual people with these problems.

G. Prognosis
1. In general the prognosis depends upon how well-developed and firmly fixed the deviation is and how motivated the person is to change.
2. Favorable prognostic signs are said to be:
   a. Seeking early treatment before complete commitment to the homosexual life-style.
   b. A sincere desire for change.
   c. Admiration for the father (in male homosexuals).
   d. Previous attempt at heterosexual intercourse.
   e. Absence of overly effeminate attitudes and mannerisms (male homosexuals).
   f. Dreams with heterosexual content.

H. Case example: A twenty-seven-year-old single man consulted a psychiatrist after he had been rejected for induction into the Army. He said that as far back as the age of ten he had been troubled with strong homosexual urges. On one occasion in the tenth grade, he developed such a strong attraction for another boy that he became "very ill" for several days and had to remain home in bed.

After graduating from art school he obtained employment as a commercial artist and had remained successfully employed in that capacity. He had a few casual acquaintances but almost no close friends. Because of his homosexual desires he purposely avoided forming friendships with other men.

His father was described as a gentle, mild-mannered man. His mother was quite the opposite, being stern, "unfeminine" and "hot-tempered." She administered the discipline in the family and, though she assumed a rather masculine role, was frequently sick in bed for one or two days every two weeks. The patient was closer to his mother than to his father.

The patient had been able to control his homosexual desires until about two years earlier when under the influence of alcohol he allowed another man to seduce him. Since that time he had a few homosexual experiences. Because of his great guilt, he has made great efforts to control his urges.

VII. Fetishism

A. Definition: Sexual excitement or gratification derived from substitution of some inanimate object, or some part of the body for a human love object. The inanimate love object is often associated with the body: for example, underwear or stockings.

B. Occurrence
1. This is a perversion peculiar to men.
2. Kinsey believed that there was a relationship between sado-masochistic behavior and fetishism.
3. Preoccupation with certain parts of the female body is called *partialism* (e.g., breasts, buttocks, legs).
4. Kleptomania in women is sometimes a source of sexual excitement, and hence, considered a fetish.

C. Theories of etiology: In addition to what has already been mentioned concerning the etiologies of other sexual deviations, the fetishist uses the fetish as a penis which then reassures him that the female also has a penis.

D. Case example: A twenty-eight-year-old married man was referred to the court psychiatric consultant after he had been arrested for touching an eighteen-year-old girl on the buttocks on two occasions on a downtown street. He admitted that he had touched between thirty to fifty girls on the buttocks, breasts, or genitalia, usually in the age range from fourteen to twenty-one, and all of them strangers. He rarely touched the same girl twice. In addition, he admitted that on three or four occasions he had made obscene propositions to the girls. He said the incidents usually occurred on his way to work or on his way home in the evening and were most apt to occur when his wife was menstruating and unavailable for sexual relationships. In all instances he denied having an erection or an orgasm but he did describe the feeling of "excitement" which he compared to the experience he had in other situations such as shooting deer. He denied other kinds of sexual problems, claiming that he got along well with his wife.

On interview he behaved very much like a schizoid person, showing a rather blunted affect and lack of verbal spontaneity. He said that on many occasions in the past he had vowed to himself to give up his deviancy but had always found it difficult to stop.

He was recommended for probationary supervision with the stipulation that he attend a psychiatric clinic.

VIII. Pedophilia

A. Definition: Pathological sexual interest in children of the same or opposite sex.

B. Occurrence: This is difficult to estimate though it is most common in adult males.

C. Theories of etiology: In addition to the etiological factors mentioned in previous sexual deviations, the male pedophile is often said to be masochistic and is frequent sexually impotent. He sees a child as a weak and approachable sexual object. Castration anxiety is said to be overwhelming. One must differentiate between the pedophile who is a sexual deviant and the person who seems to molest young children as a symptom of organic brain damage (e.g., senile deterioration).

D. Pederasty: Anal intercourse between a man and a boy.

E. Case example: Mr. I. H., a thirty-six-year-old single man, was referred to the court psychiatric consultant after he had pleaded guilty to drunkenness when he was found picking up a three-year-old boy and walking away with him. History revealed that he had been arrested on several occasions with three court appearances. Seven years earlier, he had been picked up by police for questioning after there had been complaints in a neighborhood about his frequent appearances there when there were small children around. He was released. About five years earlier, he was arrested for drunkenness and held in jail overnight. A few months later, he was arrested for disturbing the peace and on that occasion had picked up a three-year-old boy but claimed that he did nothing to him. About four years earlier, he was arrested on a charge of indecent assault when he had been arrested after picking up a four-year-old girl. He said that he was so drunk at the time that he could not remember exactly what happened. On interview, he was quiet but frank in discussing his problem and his previous court appearances. There were certain schizoid qualities to his behavior. Although he admitted that he had a problem, he was not certain as to whether or not it was sexual. He felt that his basic attraction to children was toward those who were in need of care or attention. Mental status examination did not reveal any signs of a thinking disturbance or perceptual disturbances. He was committed to a state hospital under the sexual psychopathic law.

IX. Transvestitism

A. Definition: Sexual excitation or gratification from wearing the clothing, and enacting the role of the opposite sex.
B. Occurrence
  1. It is more frequently found in males.
  2. Children sometimes dress up in the garb of the opposite sex.
  3. Some authorities say it is frequently associated with other deviations, and other describe a triad of deviancy characterized by transvestitism, fetishism, and homosexuality.
C. Theories of etiology: In addition to what has been said previously about the etiology of sexual deviancy:
  1. There is often confusion in sexual identification from the earliest years in such individuals.
  2. There may have been parental preference for a child of the opposite sex.
  3. There may have been envy of the opposite sex role.
  4. The male transvestite reacts to his castration anxiety by identifying with the phallic woman. The mother in such cases is often reported as being seductive.
  5. The female transvestite is regarded as having penis envy.
D. Prognosis is questionable because transvestites are reluctant to surrender their deviancy.
E. Treatment: Because of the reluctance on the part of the transvestite to alter his behavior, treatment has been discouraging.
F. Case example: R. U., a twenty-one-year-old married man, was referred to the court psychiatric consultant after he had pleaded guilty to a disorderly conduct charge growing out of an incident in which he was arrested in a downtown department store dressed in women's clothing and sitting in the fitting room of the dress department. Upon examination by the police physician, it was discovered that he was completely dressed in women's clothing, including padded bra, women's hose, etc. He admitted that he had dressed in women's clothing on one previous occasion about two weeks earlier. He felt his

problem was a climax to a rather deepseated sexual problem and reported that he received a thrill upon entering the women's fitting room in the department store, as he had previously when he entered the women's washroom of a downtown theatre. Just wearing the clothing stimulated him sexually. He seemed to be immature and naïve but did not show other evidences of sociopathic behavior. He was placed under probationary supervision and referred to a psychiatric clinic.

X. Transsexualism

A. Definition: A deviancy in which the person is physically normal but has a total aversion to his (or her) biological sex that dates from early childhood.

B. Difference from transvestitism: Although transsexuals frequently assume the identity of the opposite sex without surgery, they are distinguished from transvestites who derive pleasure from wearing the clothing of the opposite sex and have no desire for sex change.

C. Reconstructive surgery has been tried as a treatment technique.

D. Case example (furnished through the courtesy of Dr. Donald W. Hastings, University of Minnesota Hospitals): A 24-year-old white, single, genetic male was admitted to the hospital for transsexual surgery. He had been born in a small town in southern Minnesota and had an unusually healthy life.

He stated that from his earliest memories he had looked upon himself as a girl and that throughout his life there had never been any deviation from this. Some of these earliest memories involved dressing up in the clothes of his sister, who was two years older. He was interested exclusively in dolls, little girl's games, and playing with girls. He did not like playing with boys nor engaging in their games. His interests always were with dolls, cooking, and in high school, baton twirling. He said that he was always accepted "as a girl" by the girls in the small town in which he grew up.

By the end of grade school, he was taunted by boys for his feminine ways. It was during his midteens, while coming across descriptions of a famous case of transsexuality that it began to dawn upon him that he might be a transsexual.

He denied any overt sexual experiences of any type except for a few anal sexual experiences. He was afraid of having relationships with a genetic male "because he would quickly find out about me." He had never attempted relationships (as a man) with a genetic female—"this would disgust me." He masturbated fairly frequently and his fantasies consistently involved himself in the role of a woman, lying on his back, accepting the penis from a "straight" lover.

About four and one-half years earlier he began taking estrogens and dressing and living as a full-time woman. During this period of time there was substantial breast development and his male genitalia became "smaller" and he was unable to obtain erections. He had disgust for his penis and testicles and never felt them and kept them constantly tucked between his legs. About four years earlier he had enrolled in a beauty operators school and it was there that he met his first fellow transsexual. About two years before admission to the hospital, he had his breasts injected with liquid silicone to make them "more solid."

He was a natural blond and had never had much trouble with excessive hair or beard growth. He had a "peaches and cream" complexion and a wax application about every ten days controlled the relatively small amount of facial fuzz that he had.

In the hospital a one stage transsexual operation was performed.

XI. Exhibitionism
A. Definition: Exposure of one's body, especially the genitalia as a means of attracting sexual attention or achieving sexual excitement or gratification. The term is sometimes used in the popular sense to describe a "show-off."

B. Occurrence
   1. It is one of the more common deviations.
   2. It is usually a perversion of males. Females usually derive more pleasure from displaying other parts of their bodies.
   3. The exhibitionist often returns repeatedly to the same scene to expose himself. As a consequence, he is frequently arrested.
   4. Exhibitionistic play is common among children and is not to be considered a deviancy.

C. Theories of etiology
   1. Psychodynamically, the exhibitionist seems to be seeking reassurance for his underlying castration anxiety.
   2. A gesture of exposing may be an attempt to:
      a. Seek reassurance by having another person react to the sight of his genitalia.

   b. Seek reassurance by having other persons show fear of
      him.
   c. Seek reassurance that the female also has a penis by
      showing her what he wishes she could show him.
D. Prognosis
   1. The prognosis depends upon the exhibitionist's desire for
      change.
   2. It is also related to the severity of the deviancy.
   3. The deviancy usually ceases with aging.
E. Treatment
   1. The exhibitionist rarely seeks help voluntarily.
   2. Treatment is generally much like that listed under
      homosexuality.
F. Case example: G. J., a thirty-six-year-old married man, was
   referred to the court psychiatric consultant for evaluation
   after he had pleaded guilty to a charge of exposing himself to a
   woman in the downtown area. History indicated that he had
   begun exposing himself several months earlier, and although
   he could not give any conscious reason for the behavior, it was
   interesting to note that he had developed sexual impotence
   shortly before he experienced the first urge to expose himself.
   Although he indicated that he was worried about his impotence, he had not yet summoned up enough courage to discuss
   the matter with his personal physician. He seemed to have no
   psychological appreciation that his impotence might be
   psychogenic in origin and that this might have some relationship to his exhibitionism. Mental status examination did not
   reveal any thinking disorder or any major personality disturbance.

XII. Voyeurism (scopophilia)

A. Definition: Erotic pleasure from watching others in the
   nude, usually paying particular attention to the genitalia
   ("Peeping Tom").
B. Occurrence
   1. Sexual curiosity is universal and it is normal to be excited
      by the sight of a love object.
   2. It is probably a common deviancy although the extent is
      not known because voyeurs are quiet and unobtrusive and
      hence, rarely caught.
C. Theories of etiology
   1. See theories listed under general discussion of sexual
      deviations.

2. As with other deviations, he is seeking reassurance against castration anxieties.
3. Some see this deviation as an attempt to recreate exciting, pleasurable childhood experiences with the mother.

D. Prognosis: See the section on "Exhibitionism"
E. Treatment: See "Exhibitionism"
F. Case example: A twenty-three-year-old married man was examined by the court psychiatric consultant after he had pleaded guilty to a charge of window-peeping. He first began his voyeuristic activities in his first year of college. He estimated that he peeped in windows about once every three or four months and in that period of time had been picked up by the police on two occasions, but formally charged only once. He was a mild-mannered, frank and open individual who was basically shy and retiring but could verbalize easily about his problem. He denied any other types of sexually deviant behavior and denied that he had ever been aggressive in any sexual or asocial way. He came from an upper-middle-class family where the father was austere and emotionally removed from him. His mother was described as a seductive person who had never allowed him to have a warm relationship with his father.

Arrangements were made for him to be seen in a psychiatric clinic.

XIII. Sadism
A. Definition: Sexual excitement or gratification from inflicting physical pain on others.
B. Occurrence
1. Mild sadistic trends are common in all males.
2. Rape is a form of extreme sadism.
3. Extreme sadism is usually a psychotic symptom.
4. Sadism also refers to other acts of excessive cruelty not related to sexuality, such as beating of children.
C. Case example: Mr. Creakle, the cruel headmaster of Salemn House in *David Copperfield:* " . . .He (Creakle) then showed me the cane, and asked me what I thought of *that,* for a tooth? Was it a sharp tooth, hey? Was it a double tooth, hey? Had it a deep prong, hey? Did it bite, hey? Did it bite? At every question, he gave me a fleshy cut with it that made me writhe: so I was very soon made free of Salemn House—and was very soon in tears also."

XIV. Masochism

A. Definition: Sexual pleasure from enduring physical or psychological pain (may be inflicted by one's self or by others).

B. Occurrence

1. See "Sadism" above. Sadism and masochism often exist in the same individual.

2. Moral masochism. The seeking of humiliation and failure rather than physical pain.

C. The perversion of flagellation (erotic whipping) is one example of masochism.

XV. Sado-masochism

A. Definition: The occurrence of sadism and masochism in the same person. As noted above, these often occur together and Freud regarded masochism as sadism turned inward. The two conditions are sometimes included under the term *algolagnia*. Thus, active algolagnia is sadism and passive algolagnia is masochism.

B. Case example: A thirty-seven-year-old separated man was referred for psychiatric consultation by his attorney who was defending him in a suit filed by a woman who accused him of tying her up and beating her.

He had been aware of sado-masochistic feelings from about the age of eighteen, although he recalled pleasurable responses to being tied up by another boy at the age of eleven when they played cowboy and Indian. Since his marriage, at age twenty-one, he had gone out with a number of women. He would derive sexual pleasure from either tying up a woman or being tied up by her. He usually terminated the relationship with sexual intercourse. He says he found that women liked to be treated roughly. For the preceding five years he had intermittent difficulty with sexual impotence.

XVI. Other sexual deviations

A. Oral-anal sexual deviations

1. Fellatio (oral stimulation of the penis), cunnilingus (sexual activity in which the mouth and tongue are employed to stimulate the female genitals), and anal intercourse are not uncommon practices as part of heterosexual foreplay. Preference for these activities to the exclusion of normal heterosexual coitus is regarded as deviant.

B. Bestiality

1. Definition: Sexual gratification through intercourse with living animals.

2. Occurrence
   a. Most common in people who live in rural areas or who are socially isolated.
   b. Such people are often schizoid, mentally retarded, or overtly psychotic.
   c. It is most commonly found in adolescents, and usually involves a household pet or farm animal.
3. Case example: Mrs. J. W., a thirty-year-old, married woman, came for psychiatric treatment because of depressive symptoms. These were in part a result of a somewhat estranged relationship with her husband, who although attentive was not very sexually interested in her. During the course of her hospitalization, she became profoundly depressed when her pet dog died. At that point she revealed that on a number of occasions she had engaged in sexual relations with the dog.

C. Incest
   1. Sexual relations between members of the same family (parent-child, brother-sister, etc.).
   2. Occurrence: Although psychiatrists are aware that *incestuous feelings* are common place in their patients, they are also aware that most people erect strong defenses against them and the incest taboo is a very powerful prohibition in most cultures.
   3. Case example: A twenty-year-old college student was referred for psychiatric evaluation by a clergyman because he was sexually interested in his two teenage sisters, one of whom he had impregnated. He was a tense, anxious, nonverbal boy who bit his fingernails. He described a difficult relationship with his father. Although he had intense sexual feelings toward his two sisters, he was "scared to death" when he dated other girls.

D. Pyromania (pathological fire-setting)
   1. Definition: Erotic excitement and gratification from starting and watching fires. Sometimes the pyromaniac gets his chief pleasure from witnessing the extinguishing of the fire. Apparently, this is a reassurance that his own underlying feelings can be controlled. (The pyromaniac must be distinguished from the arsonist.)
   2. Case example: An eighteen-year-old married man was arrested for having set a number of fires in the city. Concerning the setting of the fires he indicated that he got a "thrill" or a "feeling of excitement" as he watched the fires. In

addition, he experienced some sexual gratification from setting the fires. As a matter of fact, he would set the fires in an area so that he could witness them from his place of residence and he and his wife would become sexually excited and have sexual intercourse while observing the blaze. Apart from the offense that brought him to the attention of the law, there was evidence that he had adjustment difficulties for many years. For example, obesity had been a problem with him for a long time and he gave a history of an arrest four years earlier for an assault on a two and one-half-year-old boy. He felt that he turned to homosexuality at that point because he was not able to date in high school. He denied that he had any homosexual feelings since he had been married in March of the previous year.

From clinical examination, there was no evidence that he was psychotic. In a general way, he indicated that he probably knew right from wrong and that at the time he set the first fire he knew it was wrong, but after that the rightness or wrongness of his behavior in setting additional fires did not enter his head—"it was just something I needed." There was also evidence that setting the fires relieved sexual, aggressive, and anxious feelings. At the time of the psychiatric examination in the County Jail, he was still experiencing strong desires to set fires.

E. Miscellaneous types of sexual deviations
1. Necrophilia: Sexual gratification from corpses.
2. Excretory perversions
   a. Coprophilia: Pathological sexual interest in excretions. Includes the desire to defecate on a partner or to be defecated upon.
   b. Coprophagia: A desire to eat feces.
   c. Coprolalia: The compulsive utterance of obscene words.
   d. Uralagnia: The desire to urinate on a partner or to be urinated upon.
3. Frottage: Sexual pleasure from rubbing or pressing against fully clothed members of the opposite sex. An individual so afflicted is called a fratteur. A deviation usually found in men.

XVII. Prognosis in sexual deviations, summary statement
A. In general, the prognosis depends upon the severity and the chronicity of the deviation. Where the deviation is well de-

veloped and firmly fixed and there is lack of desire for change, the prognosis is extremely poor.

B. The best prognosis seems to be in those cases where there is a relationship between the deviant behavior and some precipitating environmental stress, and among younger deviants (especially those in the adolescent years).

C. In those who are uncomfortable, anxious, or depressed as an indication that they cannot personally accept their deviancy, the response to psychotherapy is more promising. Such treatment is usually psychoanalytically oriented.

D. Since the symptom is pleasurable (ego-syntonic), it is often difficult to treat especially since the deviant seldom seeks psychiatric treatment on his own.

XVIII. Treatment, summary statement

A. There is no ideal treatment.

B. Psychotherapy is a long, drawn-out, and tedious process with sometimes doubtful results.

C. Behavioral therapy has been tried with some reported success.

D. Where the deviancy is not well fixed, response is more likely to occur in either of the above therapies.

E. Group therapy has shown some promise.

F. Environmental manipulation is sometimes of value.

G. Sometimes confinement is necessary for the protection of the community, as for example, in the pedophilic deviate who repeatedly approaches young children.

REFERENCES

Eaton, M. T., Jr., and Peterson, M. H. *Psychiatry.* 2nd ed. Flushing, New York: Medical Examination Publishing Company, 1969, chap. XIV.

Farnsworth, D. L., and Braceland, F. J., eds. *Psychiatry, The Clergy and Pastoral Counseling.* Collegeville, Minnesota: Saint John's University Press, 1969, chap. XX.

Freedman, A. M.; Kaplan, H. I., and Sadock, B. J. *Modern Synopsis of Comprehensive Textbook of Psychiatry.* Baltimore: Williams & Wilkins Company, 1972, chap. XXII.

Kolb, L. C. *Modern Clinical Psychiatry.* 8th ed. Philadelphia: W. B. Saunders Company, 1973, chap. XXVI.

Solomon, P., and Patch, V. D. *Handbook of Psychiatry.* 2nd ed. Los Altos, California: Lang Medical Publications, 1971, chap. XIX.

Oh, many a peer of England brews
livelier liquor than the muse,
and malt does more than Milton can
to justify God's ways to man.
Ale, man ale's the stuff to drink
for fellows whom it hurts to think.

Alfred E. Housman: A Shropshire Lad, 1896

Alcoholism

I. **Definition:** A personality disorder characterized by excessive use of alcohol to the point of habituation, overdependence, or addiction.

   A. Actually, several definitions have been formulated by various authorities. Some stress operational aspects while others describe causal factors.

   B. The World Health Organization regards excessive drinking to be any form of drinking which in extent goes beyond the traditional and customary use, or the ordinary compliance with the social drinking customs of the community concerned. Alcoholics are those excessive drinkers whose dependence upon alcohol has obtained such a degree that it shows a noticeable mental disturbance, or an interference with their bodily and mental health, their interpersonal relationships, their smooth and economic functioning.

   C. The *Manual on Alcoholism* of the American Medical Association (1968) gives the following definition: "Alcoholism is an illness characterized by preoccupation with alcohol and loss of control over its consumption such as to lead usually to intoxication if drinking is begun; by chronicity; by progression; and by tendency toward relapse. It is typically associated with physical disability and impaired emotional, occupational and/or social adjustments as a direct consequence of persistent and excessive use of alcohol."

D. The alcoholic has lost the power of choice in the matter of his drinking and his drinking interferes with his health, his work, his personal relationships at home. Generally, one can say that a person is an alcoholic if his drinking interferes in any way with his life.

II. Prevalence

A. Alcohol is widely used socially. Field surveys of drinking practices reveal that the prevalence rate for drinking is about 71 percent for the United States. Prevalence rates are generally higher in urban and industrial regions. Geographically, the highest prevalence is in the Middle Atlantic States (88 percent) and lowest in the East South Central Region (33 percent).

B. Today most drinking occurs in the home, whereas in the past three-quarters of all drinking occurred in bars, taverns, pubs, and restaurants.

C. Not everyone who gets drunk occasionally (or even fairly often) can be considered an alcoholic. Drinking is considered pathological only when it becomes prolonged and excessive.

D. Of the seventy to eighty million people in the United States who drink, between four and five million are said to be alcoholics (estimates vary from four and one-half million to nine and one-half million). Most of the "problem drinkers" are not found in courts, skid rows, jails, or institutions, but rather in families within the community. Since the four or five million alcoholics live in families, it is reasonable to assume that alcoholism thus directly affects sixteen to twenty million people.

E. Alcoholism accounts for about 15 percent of the first admissions to public mental hospitals.

F. Alcoholism occurs much more readily in people who have character problems or neurotic traits than it does in "normals."

G. Many alcoholics are unrecognized because their drinking is done secretly and their problem does not become manifest for a long time.

H. Some people who use alcohol to excess are not basically alcoholics; for example, the person with a manic episode who uses alcohol excessively.

I. There are about five to six times as many male alcoholics as their are female alcoholics (probably because of the different role expectancies of the two sexes). This ratio has remained fairly constant in the United States for many years even though

recent estimates suggest that the proportion of female alcoholics is increasing.

J. Much of the absenteeism problem in industry is related to
alcoholism.

K. It is also becoming an important factor in traffic accidents (in
general, courts are becoming much firmer in dealing with the
driver who is under the influence of alcohol).

III. Sociocultural factors

A. Purpose of alcohol: There are many purposes for which various sociological entities employ alcohol in specific ways. They
can be divided into <u>four general categories</u>:

1. <u>Religious</u> (e.g., wine in the Roman Catholic and Jewish
services).

2. <u>Ceremonial</u> (toasting the bride with champagne, drinking
wine at the Bar Mitzvah ceremony).

3. <u>Utilitarian:</u> As for example, cooking, medicinal purposes,
as psychic balm. It is also used at business and social functions.

4. <u>Hedonistic:</u> <u>Purely pleasurable u</u>ses. As a social lubricant
and especially for the euphoria produced.

5. These purposes can greatly influence drinking patterns
(from the *Manual on Alcoholism*, The American Medical
Association, pages 24 and 25).

B. Socioculture studies reveal low rates of alcoholism for Jews,
Chinese, and Italians. Abstinence from alcohol is uncommon
in any of these nationality groups but drunkenness is disapproved.

C. Conversely, the Irish-Americans and the French have high
rates of alcoholism. Also, studies have indicated that if a person
with a Protestant background of strict abstinence does drink,
there is relatively high likelihood that he will become a problem drinker.

D. More men than women drink and men drink larger amounts
and more frequently. This sex difference in the rate of alcoholism is sometimes explained in terms of the different role
expectancies of the two sexes. There is less social pressure
among women to drink and they are expected to drink in
fewer kinds of situations. Also, women do not have to prove
their femininity by drinking, and in addition, the negative
social sanctions against female drunkenness are much greater
than for men.

E. Studies of adolescent population show that only 2 to 6 percent of the teenage users are considered to be problem drinkers.

F. Studies of industrial populations reveal that industry numbers about two million alcoholics on its collective payroll of whom 90 percent are in the thirty-five to fifty-five age group. Some have referred to the alcoholic in the industrial setting as the "hidden half man."

IV. Etiology

A. There have been many theories proposed to explain the etiology and psychopathology of alcoholism, but the causes are not really known. Obviously, so universal a practice as alcoholic consumption would seem to indicate that alcohol satisfies some deep-seated need in human beings. Alcohol is an effective tension-reducer.

B. The causal theories may be subsumed under two chief headings: (1) pathophysiological and (2) psychological.

1. Pathophysiological theories would include any physical approach that emphasizes hereditary, metabolic, or allergic factors and largely ignores psychodynamic or cultural factors. Very few authorities subscribe to such theories.

2. Psychological theories: Most authorities believe the chief causes lie in this sphere.

C. There are certain facts which seem to be well-accepted by most authorities. First, drinking is common in our society and total abstinence rare. Second, there are many individuals who have neurotic, psychotic, or characterological difficulties, and many of them use alcohol. However, alcoholism is not common in most people who have these illnesses. Therefore, although drinking and emotional illness may be necessary conditions for the development of alcoholism, they cannot be regarded as sufficient by themselves. In addition, many people who have personality defects never use alcohol.

D. Additional facts which oppose and discredit certain commonly held views (*Manual on Alcoholism* of the American Medical Association, pages 12-13).

1. Alcohol by itself does not cause alcoholism.

2. Alcoholism does not result from drinking a particular beverage.

3. Alcoholism is not an allergic manifestation.

4. Alcoholism is not inherited.

5. Alcoholism is not due to an alcoholic personality.

E. The person who uses alcohol to excess is making an attempt at self-treatment. From a psychological point of view, the alcoholic is often said to show
   1. Emotional immaturity
   2. Emotional dependence
   3. Passivity
   4. Reduced tolerance for anxiety: anything that reduces anxiety may become a habit.
   5. Overprotective and overindulgent parental attitudes which encourage his infantile oral demands.

F. Through alcohol, one often is able to express feelings of rejection, dependency, or sexuality. This can lead to remorse and guilt afterwards and thus make it easy for the individual to drink to relieve these symptoms, too. From the psychoanalytic viewpoint:
   1. Alcoholism has been regarded as a reaction to latent homosexuality. However, many authorities now believe that the alcoholic's avoidance of relationships with the opposite sex and his preference for the company of his own sex is most likely a striving for a simple, noninvolving type of relationship.
   2. The alcoholic is regarded as having a narcissistic, premorbid personality, and under the influence of alcohol, he allows himself to return to a kind of omnipotent state, unhampered by the realities of the external world, believing that anything is possible, that he is great, and that he can do anything.

G. Conflicts at, or traumata during, the oral phase of development are also thought to be of etiological significance in alcoholism.

H. Drinking among alcoholics seems to be based largely on unconscious rather than conscious factors, and the goal of drinking seems to be to establish psychodynamic equilibrium in dealing with stresses.

I. Cultural-anthropological theories stress the influence of diverse cultural and social pressures. For example, capacity for alcoholic consumption is equated with masculinity or toughness; young men start drinking as a way of conforming to the ways of the peer group. Rates of alcoholism are higher among urban populations.

J. Alcoholism is present in virtually all socioeconomic groups.

K. In general, the underlying etiological factors for alcoholism are similar to those for psychoneurotic reactions.

L. In summary, alcoholism should probably be regarded as resulting from a complex interaction of psychological, sociocultural, and biological factors. An eclectic and empirical approach to this problem is indicated.

M. In the chronic stage, it is important to keep in mind that alcoholism should be regarded as a symptom which itself has become a disease.

V. Psychopathology

A. The alcoholic lacks some ego-strength, and like the person with character defect, he is unable to control his impulses.

B. The alcoholic shows inability to tolerate tension. This is sometimes thought to be related to his inconsistent training in dealing with reality.

C. The alcoholic has difficulty with his dependency needs. This seems related to difficulties in his very early development (the oral period, according to psychoanalytic theory).

D. The alcoholic is usually passive.

E. The alcoholic often seems socially uneasy.

VI. Symptomatology

A. The chief symptom is the excessive use of alcohol.

B. Some alcoholics have other accompanying neurotic symptoms.

C. Some alcoholics have symptoms of character defect (e.g., antisocial personality, passive-aggressive personality, inadequate personality, explosive personality).

D. Others seem to have no obvious symptom apart from the excessive drinking.

E. Toxic effects may accompany the alcoholism (see paragraph on toxic alcoholic syndromes and the chapter "Organic Brain Syndrome").

F. The defenses which seem most common among alcoholics are:
   1. Rationalization
   2. Denial
   3. Projection

G. Drinking patterns may vary. For example:
   1. Some alcoholics are "spree" or "periodic" drinkers; that is, they drink excessively for a period of time. Included in this group are the periodic alcoholics who carefully plan drinking episodes.
   2. Others are continual drinkers. Such alcoholics sip every day and, although never obviously intoxicated, are nearly always under the influence of alcohol.

H. Some authorities divide alcoholism into:
1. Essential alcoholism (addictive drinking, compulsive drinking, alcoholism simplex): Included here are those people who have drifted across the line from social drinking without any other obvious emotional problems.
2. Symptomatic alcoholism: In which the drinking is a symptom of a serious emotional illness such as anxiety reaction, depressive reaction, or schizophrenic disorder.
3. Reactive drinking: This is the type which is done in response to some particular emotional stress, as for example, the death of a loved one—the alcohol helps the individual work through his feelings of grief.
I. Seldon Bacon has given three criteria for determining the presence of alcoholism in an individual:
1. He ingests not only more alcohol, but in different ways from his appropriate associates.
2. The chronic emergence of so-called problems, especially of an intrapersonal and emotional nature, which are clearly related to this deviant use of alcohol.
3. The growing loss of rational, socially mature self-control over the ingestion of alcohol.
J. The progression into alcoholism often proceeds as follows: First, his drinking is social and masquerades as good fellowship or relaxation. Then he turns to alcohol for escape from stress and anxiety and feelings of inadequacy. Later, his self-control diminishes and his need for alcohol increases. As his control lessens, his work begins to suffer, and so also do his health, family and social relationships, and all other aspects of his life.

VII. **Toxic alcoholic syndromes:** These reactions are produced by poisoning with alcohol. They include the following:
A. Simple intoxication (nonpsychotic organic brain syndrome with alcoholism): Mainly a loss of certain inhibitions, attention disturbances, and mood changes. The mood changes may vary depending upon the personality structure. Thus, one may become depressive, euphoric, manic, paranoid, or expansive.
B. Acute alcohol intoxication: Characterized by confusion and incoordination (ataxia and slurring speech). All varieties of acute brain syndromes of psychotic proportion caused by alcohol are included here if they do not manifest features of delirium tremens, alcoholic hallucinosis, or pathological intoxication.
C. Pathological intoxication: Over-reaction to minimal amounts

of alcohol. Onset is sudden and dramatic. The person is confused, disoriented, and experiences illusions, delusions, and hallucinations. The person may become enraged, extremely anxious, depressed, maniacal, stuporous, or paranoid. Following recovery there is amnesia for the episode. It is thought to occur in people with unstable, explosive, or hysterical personality makeup. Some authorities believe that it is really a form of psychomotor epilepsy triggered by the alcohol.

D. Delirium tremens ("DT's"): An acute psychotic episode characterized by delirium, coarse tremors, and frightening visual hallucinations usually becoming more intense in the dark. It usually occurs in a chronic alcoholic after a prolonged period of drinking. The cause of the condition is not definitely known, but it is thought to be due to a metabolic disturbance. Following are the symptoms:

1. Delirium: Hallucinations are vivid, most commonly visual, and usually colorful. Tactile and olfactory hallucinations are also fairly common. Auditory hallucinations are rare. Delusions are in keeping with the hallucination. The patient is usually overactive and may be irritable, but sometimes is silly or euphoric.

2. Tremors: Tremulousness may be generalized or limited to groups of muscles.

E. Other alcoholic hallucinosis: Similar to delirium tremens but without the tremulousness. Usually follows a prolonged drinking episode. A common variety is manifest as accusatory or threatening auditory hallucinations in a state of relatively clear consciousness.

F. Korsakov's psychosis (also Korsakoff): A chronic brain syndrome characterized by amnesia, disorientation, confabulation, and peripheral neuropathy. It is associated with chronic alcoholism and results from nutritional deficiency, particularly thiamine and niacin. Symptoms are as follows:

1. Delirium of mild degree with memory and retention defects and disorientation.

2. Confabulation: The invention of an imaginary experience to fill in memory gaps.

3. Peripheral neuropathy: Most marked in the lower extremities.

G. Wernicke's syndrome: A rare encephalopathy associated with thiamine deficiency (and also niacin deficiency) and seen chiefly in chronic alcoholism. It is characterized by opthalmoplegia (most commonly nystagmus), amnesia, confabulation, ataxia, progressive deterioration, and sometimes coma. The lesions in this condition are found in the brain stem.

H. Alcoholic deterioration: Sometimes seen in persons who have had excessive alcoholic consumption for a prolonged period of time. There is gradual personality disintegration ranging from mild (emotional lability) to severe (obvious dementia). The brain damage results from a vitamin deficiency rather than from direct toxic alcoholic effect. Symptoms are in part related to the underlying basic personality structure as well as to the cerebral impairment.

I. Alcoholic paranoid state (alcoholic paranoia): This is a paranoid state which develops in a chronic alcoholic usually a male and characterized by jealousy and delusions of infidelity by the spouse. The person overuses the mechanism of projection, especially in relation to underlying homosexual strivings. Prognosis is usually poor.

VIII. Treatment

A. Treatment of the underlying personality disorder

1. Pharmacological treatment

   a. Aversion therapy: The aim of this treatment is to produce a conditioned response such that the odor or taste of alcohol will immediately lead to nausea and vomiting. The drugs used to set up such a response are emetine and apomorphine, both of which are emetics (agents that induce vomiting). This form of therapy has met with only limited success.

   b. Disulfram therapy (antabuse treatment): Following its introduction in 1948, this therapy gained ready acceptance, but it too seems to have had only limited use in the treatment of alcoholism. The drug, tetraethylthiurium disulfide, when combined with alcohol produces very distressing vasomotor symptoms. Unlike the aversion treatment, no conditioned response is established; the unpleasant effects are produced by the mixing of the antabuse and the alcohol. With this treatment, the individual must take the antabuse each day. If he stops taking the drugs for several days, he can drink alcohol without the distressing symptoms. Patients who receive this form of treatment must be in good physical health. Prior to administering the drug, special examinations of the heart, liver, and kidneys are often performed.

   c. Tranquilizing drugs: Various types of tranquilizers are

sometimes helpful in the management of alcoholism, either for facilitating psychotherapy or the mitigation of the anxiety or the symptoms of overindulgence. They are also used in the management of acute psychotic conditions related to alcoholic excesses. Among the tranquilizing medications that have been used in alcoholism are chlordiazepoxide (Librium); diazepam (Valium); chlorpromazine (Thorazine); promazine (Sparine).

2. Hospitalization is oftentimes indicated. This provides a neutral and protected environment in which psychotherapy may be attempted. It is often necessary to help the alcoholic begin a period of abstinence, as well as help him through a period of withdrawal.

3. Psychotherapy: Any psychotherapeutic approach must operate from the premise that alcoholism is a personality problem and not a moral one. The ideal treatment goal should be the elimination of the desire to drink, rather than restraint. It is also important to keep in mind that the alcoholic is usually a dependent person who often has hostile, anxious, and guilty feelings. Psychotherapy has met with only limited success, one reason being that the uncovering of conflicts produces anxiety and the alcoholic has a reduced tolerance for tension. Certain authorities emphasize the importance of "surrender" versus submission in any psychotherapeutic approach; that is, the alcoholic *must accept* the fact that he is an alcoholic and not just admit it.

4. Group therapy: Some type of group therapy is often useful in the treatment of alcoholics. Sometimes group therapy is moderated by a professional person such as a psychiatrist, clinical psychologist, or social worker.

5. Community resources
   a. Direct services to the patient
      (1) There are many agencies and organizations concerned with alcoholism.
      (2) Alcoholism Information Centers: In many communities there is a center which acts as the coordinator of available resources for the understanding and treatment of alcoholism problems.
      (3) Alcoholics Anonymous (AA): This is an informal world-wide fellowship of groups of alcoholics who

help each other to stay sober and to remain abstinent. The basic philosophy is based on twelve steps
and twelve traditions. The basic source of AA
strength is the relationship with God as the individual understands Him. For those who fit well into
formal group activity, this approach has proven effective in maintaining sobriety. Of all the available
resources, this has easily been the most helpful.
However, there are some who cannot accept this
approach, particularly those who have difficulty accepting a personal God.

(4) Industrial programs and labor union programs:
Many industries and labor unions have undertaken
comprehensive programs for alcoholic employees.

(5) Other community resources: Include many churches
and religious groups which sponsor active programs
(e.g., Calix, a group for Catholic alcoholics); the
local mental health association is also a possible
resource as well as are certain social agencies, such
as the Salvation Army.

b. Environmental
(1) Many social agencies, mental health centers, and
mental health associations can be of assistance to the
families of the alcoholic patients.
(2) Al-Anon family groups and Al-A-Teens focus on
the effect of alcoholism on the family and children.

B. Treatment of the toxic syndromes
1. Acute psychotic reactions
a. Hospitalization and withdrawal of alcohol. The withdrawal may be done gradually to mitigate the delirious
symptoms and avoid convulsions, or done abruptly.
Abrupt withdrawal is more commonly employed now
that tranquilizing drugs are available.
b. Maintaining adequate nutrition, fluid and electrolyte
intake, including the administration of intravenous
fluids and electrolytes if necessary.
c. Adequate vitamin intake, especially thiamine and niacin,
which can be administered parenterally or orally as indicated.
d. Tranquilizing drugs are often useful in the management of withdrawal symptoms. Among those that have
been used are chlorpromazine (Thorazine); promazine

(Sparine); chlordiazepoxide (Librium); diazepam (Valium).

e. Corticotropin, intramuscularly or intravenously, has been helpful in many cases of acute hallucinosis or delirium tremens.

2. Chronic psychotic reactions

a. Hospitalization is often necessary, sometimes on a permanent basis.

b. Maintaining nutrition, fluid intake, vitamin intake, etc.

c. Tranquilizing drugs may be helpful to relieve certain of the symptoms.

d. Since the brain damage is irreversible, not much definitive can be done.

IX. Prevention

A. Alcoholism is one of the four major public health concerns in the United States (along with cancer, cardiovascular disease, and mental illness).

B. There is a need to identify and discover cases of *early* alcoholism if we are to make any progress in controlling this illness. Case findings should be active rather than passive.

C. Actually, little is known about the prevention of alcoholism.

D. Research in social, psychological, and biological areas is needed.

E. The United States Government has created the National Center for Prevention and Control of Alcoholism. This is a major, federally-funded program to prevent and control alcoholism. It will work with the individual states.

X. Case reports

A. J.P.C., a thirty-eight-year-old single man, was referred to the court psychiatric consultant for evaluation after he had pleaded guilty to a charge of drunkenness, growing out of an incident in which he was arrested for behaving in a very strange manner near a neighbor's apartment building. When questioned by the police who were called, he informed the officers that he was looking for his sister who he believed was in the tree and said that she had dropped her child in a culvert and that he had retrieved the baby. He explained that his sister, while changing the baby's diaper, was snatched up into the tree. The man appeared to be intoxicated and admitted to the officers that he had been drinking. When interviewed by the psychiatric consultant, he admitted that he had been drinking excessively for years. For about one week prior to his arrest, he was aware that he was "acting screwy," that is, imagining things and that whenever he ceased drinking temporarily, he hallucinated. For example, he recalled that he believed that two men had crawled through the transom of his room at a cheap downtown hotel. This was so real to him that he phoned the police to complain. Following his arrest, he experienced other types of realistic, vivid, hallucinations. For example, he thought there were cockroaches in his cell and that the jailer was throwing ants into his cell to eat the cockroaches. In addition, he was certain that he had seen his drinking companion in jail with him and he insisted when he was bailed out by his brother that his drinking companion still remained there (which was not true).

Background history revealed that he had been arrested on approximately twenty occasions, mostly for drinking offenses, including one offense for driving while intoxicated and another for petit theft (committed while he was drinking). In addition, he had been hospitalized on three occasions at VA Hospitals for his drinking problem. He believed that his drinking had been a very serious problem for at least thirteen or fourteen years preceding the examination and he said, "It continually gets worse." He had been active with the Alcoholics Anonymous programs at various times but regarded it as a married man's organization and considered it populated by many people who were not really alcoholics.

In addition, he complained of much nervousness, uneasiness, and anxiety which he said antedated his first drinking. His Minnesota Multiphasic Personality Inventory profile revealed a high level of anxiety and indicated that he was worried, apprehensive, and tense.

He admitted to a very poor employment record over the years because of his drinking problem. He had been unemployed for the six months prior to his arrest. For approximately a year before that, he held unskilled laboring types of jobs.

This case is one of severe, chronic alcoholism in which the person also has symptoms of an anxiety neurosis. In addition, he experienced a bout of acute alcoholic hallucinosis which brought him to the attention of the police. The prognosis for this case is poor.

B. C. T., a fifty-two-year-old married woman, was admitted to the hospital at the request of her personal physician for depression and a drinking problem. Her husband, who brought her to the hospital, reported that when he had returned home from a business trip, he found his wife drunk; and she said she was unable to control her compulsive drinking. Her personal physician was summoned and arrangements were made for her admission to the hospital.

Background history revealed that she had always been a very passive person who had much difficulty with recurrent depressive feelings. On two occasions she had made suicidal attempts, once with barbiturates and on another occasion with carbon monoxide in her automobile. She had been hospitalized on at least four other occasions for psychiatric treatment.

Prominent among her symptoms while she was in the hospital were her social uneasiness and the ease with which she could feel rejected. Dependency, feelings of inferiority and inadequacy were evident also. She related that for a number of years while she was struggling with her depressive feelings and her compulsion to drink, she focused her difficulty on her husband, blaming him for her illness. About three or four years earlier, she had finally come to realize that the problem was within her and not the fault of her husband. She had tried AA on a number of occasions, but because of her passivity, she did not follow through very faithfully.

In this case, alcoholism complicates a recurrent depressive reaction. She was placed on antidepressants and psychotherapy and was referred to a local AA group for supportive help. A follow-up evaluation six months following her discharge from the hospital revealed that she had done reasonably well and had had only three minor slips where she drank a few beers over a one- or two-day period.

REFERENCES

American Medical Association. *Manual on Alcoholism*. Chicago, Ill.: American Medical Assn., 1968.

Farnsworth, D. L., and Braceland, F. J. eds. *Psychiatry, The Clergy and Pastoral Counseling*. Collegeville, Minnesota: Saint John's University Press, 1969, chap. XVII.

Jellinek, E. M. *The Disease Concept of Alcoholism*. Highland Park, N.J.: Hillhouse Press, 1960.

Keller, M. "The Definition of Alcoholism and the Estimation of Its Prevalence."

In *Society, Culture and Drinking Patterns,* edited by D.D.J. Pittman and C. R. Snyder. New York: John C. Wiley & Sons, Inc., 1962, chap. XVII.

Mendelson, J. H., ed. *Alcoholism.* Boston: Little Brown and Company, 1966.

World Health Organization, Expert Committee on Alcohol. *First Report.* Geneva: W.H.O. Technical Report Series No. 84, 1955.

I have foresworn his company hourly anytime this
two-and-twenty years, and yet I am bewitched with
the rogue's company. If the rascal have not given
medicines to make me love him, I'll be hanged:
It could be not else; I have drunk medicines.
Poins! Hal! A Plague upon you both!

Shakespeare: Henry IV

Drug Dependence

Synonyms: addiction, drug addiction

I. Definition: Marked emotional or physiological dependence on drugs to a point beyond voluntary control. (Excluded from this category are tobacco, ordinary caffeine-containing drugs, and dependence on medically prescribed drugs, so long as the drug is medically indicated and any intake is proportionate to the medical need.)

II. Introduction
  A. Terms
    1. Use: The taking of prescribed drugs under proper medical supervision.
    2. Misuse: Improper administration of drugs by a physician.
    3. Abuse: The self-administration of a drug for other than proper medical purposes.
  B. Addiction. Addiction to any drug involves three phenomenon:
    1. Tolerance: Diminishing effect with repeated use of the same dose (more and more of the drug is needed to produce effects equivalent to those experienced from the first use).
    2. Habituation: Emotional dependence upon a drug (one becomes accustomed to it but not necessarily dependent upon it).

151

3. Physical dependence: An altered physiological state such that withdrawal of the drug leads to the *abstinence syndrome.*

C. Abstinence syndrome: The withdrawal symptoms which develop when addicting drugs are withheld.
1. Withdrawal from analgesic drugs leads to:
   a. At first the patient develops yawning, rhinorrea, lacrimation, sneezing, and sweating.
   b. Next, anorexia, tremulousness, and pupillary dilatation.
   c. Later, muscular twitching, leg cramps, abdominal cramps, and backache.
   d. Last, the patient becomes extremely restless, sleepless, and shows elevated pulse and blood pressure. Diarrhea, nausea, and vomiting are often present.
   e. These intense symptoms reach their height about forty-eight hours after the last dose of the drug and remain intense for about forty-eight to seventy-two hours, gradually subsiding during the next several days.
2. Withdrawal from alcohol and hypnotic drugs may lead to:
   a. Delirium
   b. Convulsions

D. Physical Dependence Capacity (PDC): "The ability of a drug to act as a substitute for another upon which an organism has been made physically dependent; that is, to suppress abstinent phenomena that would otherwise develop after abrupt withdrawal of the original dependence-producing drug." (W.H.O. Technical Report Series No. 407, WHO Expert Committee on Drug Dependence, XVI Report, Geneva, 1969.)

III. Occurrence

A. In general, drug dependence has increased in recent years.
B. Addiction to narcotics has also increased. In April 1972, it was estimated that there were 300,000 narcotic addicts in New York City and on the basis of this, it was speculated that there were approximately 600,000 addicts in the entire United States (Freedman et al.).
C. Use of drugs among adolescents increased during the 60s, but apparently has peaked (with the possible exception of the use of marijuana).
D. Most addicts become addicted by association with an individual who is also addicted. Their life prior to addiction has usually been one of unsatisfactory or marginal adjustment.
E. Medications that reduce pain, diminish anxiety, or produce

euphoria may be taken by those who seek relief from symptoms or feelings of inadequacy.

IV. Etiology

A. Much of what was said about the etiology and psychopathology of alcoholism applies also in the case of drug dependence.

B. Drug dependence may develop after overly long administration for pain, or other type of somatic symptom, which initially was of organic origin. Such dependence has usually followed medical prescription of drugs by the individual's physician. (This is often referred to as medical addiction.)

C. Some take drugs to overcome feelings of inferiority or inadequacy.

   1. The individual who has reduced tolerance to tension, feelings of inadequacy, and who feels under stress (personal or social) may take drugs.

   2. The availability of drugs and cultural factors also may play a role here. For example, physicians are apt to use narcotics or barbiturates; housewives are most likely to use barbiturates or sedatives; jazz musicians are most apt to use marijuana.

D. Some take certain drugs mostly for the euphoric effect; for example, cocaine or marijuana.

E. Many addicts can be classified as antisocial personalities.

V. Psychopathology

A. The person who develops drug dependence has a low tension threshold and has difficulty with his dependency needs.

B. His conscience is more defective, however, since he allows himself to use drugs which, unlike alcohol, are not socially acceptable.

C. Groups:

   1. Antisocial personalities: Persons in this group become addicted chiefly through contact with others who are addicts.

     a. Are usually immature, hostile, aggressive people.

     b. They take drugs primarily for "the kicks."

   2. Neurotic persons: Persons in this group take drugs to relieve physical or psychological symptoms.

   3. Painful physical illness: Drugs had been prescribed over an extended period and dependence on the drugs persisted after the illness had ceased.

D. Some authorities believe that there is absence of a strong father-figure in the developmental histories of people who become addicts.

VI. Types of dependency-producing drugs: The following are some of the drugs on which people can become dependent.

   A. Narcotics: Included in this group are opium, morphine, heroin, and their derivatives as well as synthetic substitutes for narcotics.

      1. Morphine

         a. The majority of such addicts use to adjust to pain of organic origin or discomfort of emotional origin.

         b. With the individual's increase in tolerance come irritability and intellectual inefficiency.

         c. Some chronic users deteriorate and show economic and moral decline. Many get into legal difficulties because of their addiction; for example, they may be arrested for illegal purchase of the drug or for stealing to get money to buy the drug.

      2. Other opium derivatives

         a. Heroin: can be obtained only illegally. The most addicting of all drugs and is said to be the most difficult addiction to treat.

         b. Codeine: the addiction probability is quite low with this drug.

         c. Dilaudid and other drugs are also addicting.

      3. Demerol: Is a synthetic analgesic. It is not chemically related to morphine but it is addicting.

      4. Cocaine

         a. Has a limited use in medical practice.

         b. Is taken either by hypodermic injection or by "sniffing" (sniffing snow).

         c. Produces euphoria and increased motor activities.

         d. Somatic hallucinations (including the "cocaine bug") are sometimes experienced.

   B. Sedative drugs

      1. Bromides

         a. Bromides were used extensively for many years until the introduction of barbiturates about a generation ago. Barbiturates and the newer sedatives have replaced them as drugs prescribed for sleeping, and the tranquilizers have replaced them as relievers of anxiety.

         b. The effects of bromides are similar to those of barbiturates.

    c. Skin rash (drug dermatitis) may develop in people who have been taking bromides for long periods of time.

    d. The blood bromide level will be elevated in people who have been taking toxic doses.

  2. Barbiturates

    a. Barbiturates were very commonly prescribed in the past for various types of neurotic symptoms. They are still fairly widely prescribed for sedation, although the recent introduction of nonbarbiturate sedatives has reduced their use.

    b. The most common users have been neurotics who have symptoms of anxiety, depression, or insomnia.

    c. Most users have passive-aggressive personality traits and show conflict about aggressive, sexual, and dependency strivings.

    d. These drugs produce relaxation and a sense of well-being (i.e., sedation). Such effects are very similar to the effects of alcohol.

    e. Although most persons addicted to barbiturates can be withdrawn rather abruptly, on rare occasions abrupt withdrawal may produce convulsions or a toxic delirium.

  3. Nonbarbiturate sedatives: Some people have become dependent on some of the newer nonbarbiturate sedatives. Among these are: Placidyl, Doriden; Noludar.

C. Minor tranquilizers

  1. See chapter on "Treatment In Psychiatry" for characteristics of this group of drugs which produce calmness and relaxation.

  2. Dependency on some of them has been reported: Meprobamate (Equanil; Miltown); Chlordiazepoxide (Librium); and Diazepam (Valium). Addiction does not develop with major tranquilizers (such as the Phenothiazine group).

D. Central Nervous System Stimulants (CNS): especially amphetamine, methamphetamine and their derivatives.

  1. These were widely used before the introduction of the modern antidepressant drugs. They were prescribed to relieve fatigue and depression, or to control appetite or to produce wakefulness in those who had to perform tasks of long duration.

  2. These drugs are now under much closer governmental

supervision because of the widespread abuse that developed.

3. These drugs are stimulants and produce euphoria.
4. Dependence sometimes develops in those who take for weight control or to stay awake.
5. Sometimes those who are dependent on sedatives for sleep take these during the day to stay awake.
6. Acute paranoid psychosis may develop in people who abuse this group of drugs.

E. Hallucinogenic drugs
   1. Among these are lyseric acid/diethylamide (LSD); mescaline (Peyote) from cactus; psilocybin, from mushroom; dimethyltryptamine (DMT); STP; morning glory seeds; nutmeg, and stramonium.
      a. Most produce a reaction similar to hypomania and schizophrenic withdrawal (preoccupation with own thoughts and perceptions).
      b. These drugs can lead to serious psychological damage.
      c. Some of the adverse affects that have been reported from LSD usage are:
         (1) Long-term psychotic reactions.
         (2) Panic ("bad trip") from a reaction to the hallucinatory experiences.
         (3) Serious injury and even death from the delusional experiences (feelings of omnipotence or the feeling that one can fly, etc.)
         (4) Long-term intellectual and emotional disorientation.
         (5) Flashback phenomenon: a reexperiencing of a "trip" without further use of the drug.
   2. Marijuana
      a. This drug is not used in modern medicine.
      b. The leaf grows wild in most parts of the United States.
      c. It has been used in the United States since about 1920, and was first used by members of deprived socioeconomic groups, but lately has been used increasingly by members of the middle and affluent classes.
      d. It is symptomatic of intrapsychic as well as social problems.
      e. There is some evidence to suggest that it is associated with criminal activity although the drug itself does not produce criminal activity.

    f. Like cocaine, it produces euphoria and increased motor activity.

    g. True tolerance does not develop and thus abrupt withdrawal does not produce physiological disturbances (withdrawal symptoms). However, it is considered an habituating drug.

    h. Continued use produces apathy and indifference.

    i. Some musicians who take it claim that it lengthens time and thus allows them to perform better.

F. Glue sniffing

    1. Found among some children who are depressed, passive-aggressive, and have histories of delinquencies.

    2. Physiological dependence does not develop.

    3. Other sniffing: gasoline vapor, pure toluene, ether, lighter fluid.

VII. Treatment

A. Of the underlying personality disorder.

    1. This is usually extremely difficult because the addict, like the alcoholic, has reduced tolerance for tension.

    2. Psychotherapy is of help in many cases. Support and reassurance are important.

    3. Group therapy, including groups similar to Alcoholics Anonymous, has been of help to many addicts.

    4. The U.S. Public Health Service has established a special hospital for the study and treatment of addiction.

B. Of the drug dependence. General principles of treatment:

    1. Withdrawal of the drug

        a. In the past narcotic addicts were often withdrawn in one of three ways:

            (1) Abrupt withdrawal: Stopping the drug immediately.

            (2) Rapid withdrawal: Withdrawal of the drug over a period of seven to fourteen days.

            (3) Gradual withdrawal: Withdrawing the drug over a period of thirty or more days.

        b. Presently most drug dependent people are withdrawn fairly abruptly utilizing the principles outlined under supportive treatment below.

    2. Supportive treatment

        a. Judicious use of tranquilizers (e.g., Meprobamate, Librium, Valium, Sparine, or Thorazine), especially during the withdrawal period.

b. Sedatives may be prescribed to aid sleep (e.g., the milder, nonaddicting, nontoxic types of sedatives such as Chloral Hydrate and Dalmane.)

c. Insulin in small doses before meals is often a good stimulant to appetite.

d. Adequate fluid intake and diet should be maintained.

e. Such persons often need "attention" more than other patients. It is important to maintain a therapeutic, supportive, and reassuring attitude. One should avoid being judgmental or moralistic.

C. Methadone (Dolophine): This is a treatment for addiction to opiate and opiatelike agents.

1. Methadone substitution: In this approach the addict is stabilized on a dose of Methadone, given orally, after which he is progressively withdrawn from the drug over a period of a few days.

2. Methadone maintenance: In this method, the administration of the Methadone is maintained indefinitely.

D. Rehabilitation of the drug-dependent person must be regarded as a long-term management problem.

VIII. Prognosis

A. Ordinarily the prognosis is considered to be poor.

B. Relapses are common.

C. However, given someone who is well motivated and willing to regard his problem as a long-term one that must be dealt with consistently over a protracted period of time, the frequency of relapses can be reduced and the period of abstinence from the drugs can be lengthened.

IX. Case reports

A. A case of medical addiction: Mrs. J., a forty-year-old housewife, had suffered with migraine headaches since puberty. They had gradually increased in frequency and severity during the years. At the age of thirty she began taking codeine for the relief of the headaches. For a few years this gave some relief but for the previous five years she had been taking demerol (a synthetic narcotic drug) in increasingly larger doses. At the time of admission to the hospital she was using 500-600 mgm. of demerol per day (usual dose is 50 mgm.).

She was always very dependent on her mother. Even after her marriage she never lived farther away from her mother than one block. She had always had a reduced tolerance of any kind of discomfort; for example, she required medication for painful menses, sinusitis, etc.

Although she was successfully withdrawn from demerol by the Rapid method during her hospitalization, she was never fully able to face her problems of underlying dependency and unexpressed hostility. One month after discharge she was again beginning to take demerol for her headaches.

In the foregoing case, note that the patient began taking drugs for a psychosomatic illness (migraine) and that she had reduced tolerance of discomfort, was very dependent, and showed inability to express hostile feelings.

B. A case of drug abuse from self administration: Mr. D. S., a twenty-three-year-old single male caucasian, was referred to the court psychiatric consultant for evaluation after he had been placed in the Workhouse for (1) driving after suspension of his license and (2) driving under the influence of drugs. These offenses occurred while he was awaiting trial on a charge of aggravated robbery.

He received an undesirable discharge from the Marine Corps "at my own request," centering around his possession and use of marijuana. In addition to this, he said he had once been court-martialed for disrespect to a staff noncommissioned officer and had received minor disciplinary actions for two other offenses. Concerning his use of drugs, he said that he was first "turned on" by marijuana about three years earlier while serving in the Marines. From then until the time of the arrest which brought him to the attention of the court consultant, he admitted using drugs extensively. He had used LSD and other hallucinogenic drugs but gave these up after he began to have "bad trips" and "flashbacks" from them. He said that he had been hospitalized in Okinawa for a four-day period to withdraw him from hallucinogenic drugs and had also suffered some minor withdrawal symptoms when he was jailed for the current offenses. Chiefly, he had been "mainlining" heroin, although he also used cocaine. Throughout all of this time of his abuse of drugs, he had never tried to stop marijuana although he said that for periods of up to one or two months during the preceding four years he had been able to remain off of other drugs. He also admitted that he had used "speed" intravenously. He said that his habit was costing him from $100 to $120 per day.

Mental status examination revealed him to be somewhat anxious and superficial and he seemed to try to impress the examiner with his need to be released from incarceration. He admitted feeling depressed in the past when his freedom was restricted and also sometimes from the bad effects of drugs. Although he was lucid, appropriate, and free of psychotic mentation, he said that he was aware of paranoid ideation at times in the past when he was on drugs. He also admitted having hallucinatory experiences on LSD, mescaline, and on one occasion from "Panama Marijuana." In all of these instances he had pleasant, colorful visions, and auditory sensations. Mostly his early trips were pleasant, but later the trips became paranoid and would last up to five hours.

Needle scars were evident over the antecubital areas of both arms.

Treatment in a hospital setting was recommended for his drug dependency problem.

REFERENCES

Farnsworth, Dana L., and Braceland, F. J., eds. *Psychiatry, the Clergy and Pastoral Counseling.* Collegeville, Minnesota: Saint John's University Press, 1969, chap. XVIII.

Freedman, A. M.; Kaplan, H. I.; and Sadock, B. J. *Modern Synopsis of Comprehensive Textbook of Psychiatry.* Baltimore: Williams & Wilkins Company, 1972, chap. XXI.

Kolb, L. C. *Modern Clinical Psychiatry.* 8th ed. Philadelphia: W. B. Saunders Company, 1973, chap. XXVII.

World Health Organization, Expert Committee on Drug Dependence. Geneva: Technical Report Series No. 407, XVI Report, 1969.

Mankind is made up of inconsistencies,
  and no man acts invariably up to his predominant character.
The wisest man sometimes acts weakly and the
  weakest sometimes wisely.

Lord Chesterfield: LETTER TO HIS SON,
April 26, 1748

Transient Situational Disturbances
Special Symptoms, Behavior Disorders, and Other Conditions

I. **Introduction:** Transient situational disorders are more or less transient in character and appear to represent an acute reaction to an overwhelming environmental stress in an individual without evident underlying mental disorder. The symptoms subside when the stress diminishes.

II. **Types:** Disorders in this category are classified according to the patient's developmental stage as follows:

  A. Adjustment reaction of infancy: These are transient reactions occurring in infants growing out of the infant's interaction with parental figures or other important figures in his life. Examples are excitability, apathy, sleep disturbances, feeding disturbances.

  B. Adjustment reaction of childhood: Included are the transient reactions of children to some particular internal emotional strife or immediate situational problems.

  C. Adjustment reaction of adolescence: Those transient disturbances of adolescence which are expressions of emancipatory struggles are included here.

  D. Adjustment reaction of adult life: This refers to a reaction to a difficult situation or environmental factor of recent origin in someone who has no apparent evidence of underlying serious personality problems. It can be manifested as any one of a number of symptoms, as for example, low morale, unconventional behavior, anxiety, alcoholism, etc. Some of these reactions, if untreated, may progress into one of the typical psychoneurotic reactions.

E. Adjustment reaction of late life: Under this group are included those reactions of later life.

SPECIAL SYMPTOMS

I. **Introduction:** This category is reserved for the occasional case where a particular symptom is the single, chief expression of underlying psychopathology. This is not to be used in those instances where symptoms are associated with other kinds of psychiatric illness, such as the psychogenic psychoses or the organic brain syndromes.

II. **Examples**
   A. Speech disturbance
   B. Specific learning disturbance
   C. Tic
   D. Other psychomotor disorder
   E. Disorder of sleep
   F. Feeding disturbance
   G. Enuresus
   H. Encopresis
    I. Cephalalgia
   J. Other special symptoms

BEHAVIOR DISORDERS OF CHILDHOOD AND ADOLESCENCE

I. **This category** is reserved for disorders occurring in childhood and adolescence that are more stable, internalized, and resistant to treatment than transient situational disturbances, but less so than psychoses, neuroses, and personality disorders.

II. **Classification:** Included under this group of disorders are the following:
   A. Hyperkenetic reaction of childhood (or adolescence): Characterized by overactivity, restlessness, distractibility, and short attention span.
   B. Withdrawing reaction of childhood (or adolescence): Characterized by seclusiveness, detachment, sensitivity, shyness,

timidity, and general inability to form close personal relationships.

C. Overanxious reaction of childhood (or adolescence): Characterized by chronic anxiety, excessive and unrealistic fears, sleeplessness, nightmares, and exaggerated autonomic responses.

D. Run-away reaction of childhood (or adolescence): Characterized by running away from home for a day or more without permission in response to a threatening situation.

E. Unsocialized aggressive reaction of childhood (or adolescence): Characterized by overt or covert hostile disobedience, quarrelsomeness, physical and verbal aggressiveness, vengefulness, and distrustfulness.

F. Group delinquent reaction of childhood (or adolescence): Characterized by the acquisition of values and behavior or skills of a delinquent peer group or gang.

G. Other reaction of childhood (or adolescence).

CONDITIONS WITHOUT MANIFEST PSYCHIATRIC DISORDER AND NONSPECIFIC CONDITIONS

I. **This category** is for those conditions occurring in individuals who would be considered psychiatrically normal, but have problems severe enough to warrant examination by a psychiatrist. These conditions may either become or precipitate a recognizable psychiatric disorder.

II. **Classification**
    A. Marital maladjustment
    B. Social maladjustment (cultural shock)
    C. Occupational maladjustment
    D. Dyssocial behavior: This category is for those individuals who are not classifiable as antisocial personalities, but are predatory and follow more or less criminal pursuits, such as racketeers, dishonest gamblers, prostitutes, and dope peddlers.
    E. Other social maladjustments

DYSSOCIAL BEHAVIOR

I. **Introductory comment:** Individuals in this group show disregard for the usual social and moral codes and often come in conflict with them as the result of having lived all or most of their lives in an abnormal moral environment.

II. Occurrence

A. These individuals come largely from the lower socioeconomic group.

B. Such reactions are much less common than antisocial reactions.

III. Etiology and psychopathology

A. These individuals lack a well-developed superego or conscience.

B. They are said to be more passive than individuals who show antisocial reactions.

C. The family constellation is thought to show far more psychopathology.

D. In general, what was mentioned under "etiology" and "psychopathology" in the chapter on "Antisocial Reactions" applies here.

IV. Symptomatology

A. In general, people in this group attempt gratification of all types of instinctual needs.

B. Included in this group are some sexually promiscuous people, gamblers, and members of gangs.

V. Case example: A. L. A., a twenty-year-old single Puerto Rican, was

referred to the court psychiatric consultant for examination after he had pleaded guilty to a disorderly conduct charge growing out of an incident in which he forcibly entered a girl's apartment, pushed her around, and threatened her with a knife. Shortly before doing this, he had forced his way into a party in the same apartment building even though he was not invited and did not know any of the people. His record indicated four previous arrests, all in Spanish Harlem in New York (these offenses were for truancy, carrying equipment to inject narcotics, petit larceny, etc.).

Background history revealed that he had been born in Puerto Rico but had spent most of his life in the Spanish Harlem section of New York City, where he grew up in association with boys who expected delinquent behavior from everyone in the group. His early childhood was marked by emotional deprivation and rejection on the part of his father. His mother had died when he was about three years old. His job record was characterized by either discharges for unsatisfactory performance or termination when he did not feel like working.

On examination he was without anxiety, guilt, or remorse. He did not regard himself as having any nervous problems and did not show any evidence of thinking disturbances or delusions. He admitted to using alcohol to excess at times, and when he drank, he was easily provoked and got mad. He could discuss the four arrests in New York and blamed this on "hanging around with the wrong kids." He did not seem to show any concern that his behavior displayed manifest disregard for the usual social codes of other people.

He was given a workhouse sentence, but a portion of this was suspended and he was placed under probationary supervision.

REFERENCE

American Psychiatric Association. *Diagnostic and Statistical Manual of Mental Disorders*. 2d ed. Washington, D.C., 1968. Seventh printing, July 1974.

Functional Psychoses

Psychoses not attributable to physical conditions listed previously
(295-298)

  I. Definition: psychotic disorders which are not caused by any known
  physical condition. In previous classifications they have been listed
  as disorders of psychogenic origin.

 II. Classification: It should be recalled that under the present classifi-
  cation only the functional psychoses are included in this group.
  The formal heading is: "Psychoses Not Attributable to Physical
  Conditions Listed Previously." Psychotic reactions of organic
  origin are classified under "Psychoses Associated with Organic
  Brain Syndromes."

III. Psychoses not attributable to physical conditions listed previously
  (295-298)
  A. Schizophrenia (295): A group of disorders characterized by
    disturbances in thinking, mood, and behavior.
    1. Schizophrenia, simple type: Characterized chiefly by a slow
      and insidious reduction of external attachments and in-
      terests by apathy and indifference.
    2. Schizophrenia, hebephrenic type: Characterized by disor-
      ganized thinking, shallow and inappropriate affect, un-

predictable giggling, silly, regressive behavior and mannerisms, frequently by hypochondriacal complaints. Delusions and hallucinations, if present, are transient and not well organized.

3. Schizophrenia, catatonic type:
   a. Excited: Characterized by excessive, and sometimes violent, motor activity and excitement.
   b. Withdrawn: Characterized by stupor, mutism, negativism, and waxy flexibility.

4. Schizophrenia, paranoid type: Characterized primarily by the presence of persecutory or expansive delusions.

5. Acute schizophrenic episode: Characterized by an acute onset of schizophrenic symptomatology often associated with confusion, perplexity, ideas of reference, emotional turmoil, dreamlike association and excitement, depression or fear.

6. Schizophrenia, latent type: Characterized by clear symptoms of schizophrenia but without history of psychotic, schizophrenic episodes. Disorders sometimes designated as incipient, prepsychotic, pseudoneurotic, pseudopsychopathic, borderline schizophrenia, or chronic undifferentiated are sometimes categorized here.

7. Schizophrenia, residual type: A category of patients who have suffered a psychotic schizophrenic episode but who are no longer psychotic.

8. Schizophrenia, schizo-affective type: Characterized by a mixture of schizophrenic and affective symptoms.
   a. Schizophrenic, schizo-affective type, excited (schizophrenic symptoms plus elation).
   b. Schizophrenia, schizo-affective type, depressed (schizophrenic symptoms with depression).

9. Schizophrenia, childhood type: This category is for those cases in which the schizophrenic symptoms appear before puberty. Autism, atypical, withdrawn behavior, and inability to develop identity are characteristics of this illness.

10. Schizophrenia, chronic, undifferentiated type: A category for those who show mixed schizophrenic symptoms and who present definite schizophrenic thought, affect, and behavior not classifiable under the other types.

11. Schizophrenia, other: A category for any type of schizophrenia not previously described.

B. Major affective disorders (affective psychoses—296): Characterized by a single disorder of mood, either extreme depression or elation.

1. Involutional melancholia: A disorder with onset in the involutional period and characterized by worry, anxiety, agitation, and severe insomnia.

2. Manic-depressive illness (manic-depressive psychosis): This disorder is marked by severe mood swings and a tendency to remission and recurrence.

    a. Manic-depressive illness, manic type (manic-depressive psychosis, manic type): Characterized by the occurrence of manic-episodes (elation, irritability, talkativeness, flight of ideas, and accelerated speech and motor activity).

    b. Manic-depressive illness, depressed type (manic-depressive psychosis, depressed type): Characterized by the recurrence of depressive episodes (depressive mood, mental and motor retardation).

    c. Manic-depressive illness, circular type (manic-depressive psychosis, circular type): Characterized by both depressive and elated episodes.

        (1) Manic-depressive illness, circular type, manic.
        (2) Manic-depressive illness, circular type, depressed.

3. Other major affective disorders (affective psychosis, other): Major affective disorders for which a more specific diagnosis has not been made are included here. It is also for "mixed" manic-depressive illness in which manic and depressive symptoms appear almost simultaneously. It does not include *psychotic depressive reaction,* or *depressive neurosis.*

C. Paranoid states (297): Psychotic disorders in which a delusion, generally persecutory or grandiose, is the essential abnormality. They are usually without hallucinations or schizophrenic behavior.

1. Paranoia: A very rare psychotic disorder characterized by an elaborate, well-systematized, complex, intricate, logical, and well-fixed delusional system but with relatively good preservation of the remainder of the personality.

2. Involutional paranoid state (involutional paraphrenia): A paranoid psychosis with initial onset of delusion formation in the involutional period (late middle life).

3. Other paranoid states: An ill-defined group of reactions characterized by paranoid delusions which lack the logical systematization seen in paranoia but which do not show the

regression and deterioration found in paranoid schizophrenia (this is a residual category for paranoid psychoses
which are not classifiable elsewhere).

D. Psychotic depressive reaction (reactive depressive
psychoses—298.0): A psychosis distinguished by depressive
mood attributable to some experience and without a history of
repeated depressions or cyclothymic mood swings.

The classification and descriptions of conditions in this chapter closely
follow those given in the *Diagnostic and Statistical Manual of Mental Disorders,* Second Edition, Seventh Printing, 1974.

Affective Disorders

I. Introduction

A. The term *affective disorder* is a general one and refers to a personality disorder in which the fundamental disturbance is in the mood (affect).

B. The mood changes—depression or elation—differ from normal mood swings chiefly in degree and duration. The change may be without apparent cause, seem disproportionate, or persist too long.

C. Any disturbances in thought or behavior are appropriate to the mood.

II. Clinical types

A. Cases of affective disorders really fall along a continuum, varying from mild, short-lived, subclinical depressions and elations on one end, to the severe delusional depressions and delirious manias on the other.

B. Included in the discussion of these disorders are the following:
1. Manic-depressive illness
2. Involutional melancholia
3. Psychotic-depressive reaction (reactive-depressive psychosis)
4. Depressive neurosis

C. It should be kept in mind that only manic-depressive illness and involutional melancholia belong to the group, Major affective disorders (Affective psychoses), in the DSM-II. Depressive neurosis, as indicated earlier, is a type of neurotic disturbance, and psychotic-depressive reaction is classified separately. However, all of these are discussed in this chapter because they are mood disturbances.

III. Degrees of depression
A. Grief (bereavement): A normal, appropriate, affective sadness in response to a recognizable external loss. It is realistic and appropriate to what has been lost; it is self-limiting and gradually subsides. It seldom leads to serious disorder in one's personal life.
B. Neurotic depression: The etiologic factor is less obvious than in normal grief, or the depression is more severe, or persists unduly long. Oftentimes, the external situation which occasions the reaction is more a precipitating event rather than a causal factor. The individual usually realizes he is responding excessively but does not recognize the underlying cause.
C. Psychotic depression: The depression is so profound that the patient loses contact with reality, develops delusions, and frequently is a serious suicidal risk.

IV. Symptoms common to any depression
A. There are certain symptoms that usually are found in any type of depression. These vary according to the type and severity of the depression.
B. Symptoms
  1. Sleep disturbance: This may be manifested as difficulty in falling asleep, difficulty in staying asleep, or early morning awakening.
  2. Appetite disturbance: This may be diminished interest in food, absence of appetite, or refusal to eat for delusional reasons.
  3. Often the individual feels better in the evening than in the morning (there is no good explanation for this).
  4. Somatic symptom: This may be manifested as a mild physiological response of any body system, hypochondriacal preoccupation, definite physical symptoms, or somatic delusions. Often it is the somatic symptom which first concerns the patient and leads him to seek medical examination.

V. Descriptive types of depression

A. Aside from the official diagnostic classification of the various depressive reactions, certain clinical types of depression are often described.

B. Clinical types of depression
1. Overt depressions
   a. Retarded depression (as seen in certain depressive neuroses and in some of the depressive phases of manic-depressive reactions).
   b. Agitated depression (as seen in classical involutional melancholia).
   c. Ideational (as seen in some depressive neuroses).
2. Covert (masked) depressions
   a. Hypochondriacal (in this type, physical symptoms disguise the underlying symptom). This type may also be diagnosed hypochondriacal neurosis (see chapter on "Neuroses").
   b. Neurasthenic (here the major complaints are exhaustion, fatigue, and weakness. This is sometimes diagnosed neurasthenic neurosis or neurasthenia (see chapter on "Neurosis").

VI. Suicide

A. Introductory comments
1. Since the possibility of suicide frequently is raised in the depressive reactions of all types, it is considered here.
2. However, it should be kept in mind that suicide is not exclusively limited to people with such diagnoses. Nearly everyone has had death wishes about himself or even suicidal thoughts.
3. A fairly large number of people have at certain times in their lives contemplated suicide either in a passive or an active way. However, the number of suicidal attempts is fortunately much smaller than the number who have contemplated it, and the percentage of successful suicide is fortunately even much smaller. It is variously estimated that attempts are five to fifty times more common than successes (the most common estimate seems to be ten attempts for every successful suicide).

B. Occurrence
1. Suicide is the tenth major cause of death in the United States.
2. Incidence: About ten to twelve per hundred thousand population in the United States.

3. Sociocultural influences: It is less common in Catholic countries, such as Ireland, and more common in Japan, Germany, Denmark, and Switzerland.
4. Cultural attitudes toward suicide, death, and afterlife seem to play a role.
5. Some studies indicate that it is rare for people to make more than one suicide attempt.
6. Although more attempts are made by women in the United States, more men are successful.

C. Psychodynamic factors
1. Most authorities believe that suicide rarely results from a single cause. Several factors may be opperant in an accumulative way.
2. Any serious loss may be a possible etiological factor: for example, loss of a loved one, a job, money, health, beauty, independence.
3. Sometimes, in a depressed person, the anniversary date of an important event (e.g., the death of a loved one) may initiate a suicidal attempt.
4. Karl Menninger regards suicide as self-murder.
5. Schneidman and Farberow have classified people who commit suicide into four general groups:
   a. Those who view suicide as a means to a better life or as a means of saving reputation.
   b. Those who are psychotic and commit suicide in response to delusions or hallucinations.
   c. Those who commit suicide out of revenge against a loved person.
   d. Elderly and infirm people who use suicide as a release from pain.
6. What prods a person from contemplation to action is not really known.
7. Some feel suicide attempts are motivated by:
   a. A wish for revenge
   b. Feelings of hopelessness
   c. Fantasies of reunion (anniversary suicide). Thus, suicide contains a wish to kill as well as a wish to die. Hostility toward a rejecting person, presumed or actual, may motivate the individual to attempt to kill himself, and thus make the rejecting person guilty.

D. Danger Signs
1. History of previous suicidal attempts or threats
2. Suicide note

        3. Psychotic reactions with suspiciousness, paranoid delusions, or panic
        4. Chronic illness
        5. Alcoholism or drug dependency
        6. Advancing age, especially in men
        7. Recent surgery or childbirth
        8. Hypochondriasis
        9. Homosexuality
  E. Evaluation of suicidal risks. When estimating a person's suicidal potential the following questions are helpful:
        1. Have you thought of suicide?
        2. Have you thought of what way you would take your life?
        3. Have you already made preparations?

DEPRESSIVE NEUROSIS

Synonyms: depressive reaction; reactive depression, neurotic depression

   I. Definition: A pathological state of sadness in which the etiological factor is less obvious than in normal grief, or the depression is more severe, or persists unduly long. Oftentimes, the external situation which occasions the reactions is more a precipitating event than a causal factor. The individual usually realizes he is responding excessively but does not recognize the underlying cause.

  II. Occurrence: Depression, either as a single symptom or as part of other symptom complexes, is extremely common in psychiatric practice. It is also commonly found in general medical practice, although the depressive symptoms are sometimes not readily recognized or are not so obvious. (Covert depression often goes unrecognized.)

 III. Symptomatology
    A. See previous section.
    B. The onset is frequently related to a loss or failure of some type and may be sudden or slow in developing.
    C. In general, depressive neurosis is characterized by difficulty in concentration or thinking, depressed mood, and psychomotor retardation. (A generalized reduction of physical and emotional responses; e.g., loss of interest or drive, diminished ambition, reduced libido.)
    D. Sleep and appetite are disturbed, and the patient usually complains of some somatic symptom.

E. If the depression is severe, there may be suicidal preoccupation.

IV. Psychopathology

A. Premorbid personality: Usually occurs in an individual with a history of previous neurotic traits. Often such people have been described as shy, sensitive, pessimistic, dependent, and worrisome.

B. Fundamentally, there is a loss of self-esteem. This is related to:

1. Damaged *self-image*, which usually develops in an unfavorable family relationship.

2. Disparity between the *superego* value system and the individual's behavior leading to guilt.

3. An overly exaggerated *ego-ideal* which leads to the development of feelings of inadequacy and inferiority.

4. Poor coordination of other *ego-functions* with consequent discrepancy between the abilities and the ego-ideal.

C. The presence of ambivalent feelings. (The coexistence of two opposing feelings toward the same individual or object. Such feelings may be conscious or unconscious.) Thus, in depressive neurosis, there are both affection and hostility toward a desired person or object.

D. The depressed person feels guilty about his hostile feelings.

E. Because of the guilt, there is introjection of hostile feelings. The individual directs unacceptable aggressive and hostile impulses toward himself, that is, toward the introjected object or person within himself. This leads to feelings of unworthiness, guilt feelings, and depression. (See "Adjustive Patterns.")

V. Prognosis: Spontaneous remission is usual. Treatment usually reduces the duration of a given episode. Relapses may occur.

VI. Treatment

A. Although spontaneous remission is common, psychotherapy is the treatment of choice. This should include emotional support, reassurance, understanding, tolerance of the individual's dependency and acceptance of his complaints without becoming angry, as well as environmental manipulation.

B. Antidepressant medications are usually very helpful. Sometimes tranquilizers are indicated for the anxiety that is frequently present in depressive neurosis. Sedatives at bedtime are often necessary to relieve the insomnia problem.

C. Sometimes electroshock therapy is used if the depression is severe or refractory to other types of treatment.

D. Oftentimes a combination of these approaches is necessary.

VII. Case example: Mrs. S., a thirty-five-year-old housewife, was admitted to the hospital complaining of nausea, vomiting, crying, and depression. Her symptoms had begun four months earlier following an incident which should have made her feel hostile to her husband. However, because of guilt related to an extramarital affair a few years earlier, she was unable to express her hostile feelings and these became redirected against herself and produced the depressive symptoms. On admission, she appeared depressed and cried rather easily when discussing her illness and her husband. There was no obvious psychomotor retardation, but she did complain of some difficulty in concentration. In the hospital, she ate poorly and had difficulty sleeping. She responded promptly to treatment and has remained free of symptoms for several years.

In the foregoing, the patient showed symptoms common to most depressions, namely, depressed mood, difficulty in concentration, appetite and sleep disturbance, and somatic symptoms.

MANIC-DEPRESSIVE ILLNESS

Synonyms: manic-depressive reaction; manic-depressive psychosis

I. Definition: Psychotic reactions characterized by severe mood swings—elation and depression—and a tendency to remission and recurrence. They do not progress to a state of deterioration.

II. History
  A. Melancholia and mania were described in ancient times and were differentiated from some of the other psychoses.
  B. Kraepelin proposed the present name.

III. Prevalence
  A. The exact prevalence of these disorders is not really known. (Estimates vary between 5 percent and 15 percent of patients admitted for psychiatric disorders.)
  B. It is twice as common among women (at least for hospitalized cases).
  C. The incidence has probably decreased during this century.
  D. The incidence is said to be higher among Irish and Jewish people and lower among the Scandinavian and Northern European peoples.
  E. The worldwide incidence is about three to four per one thousand.
  F. Onset is usually between the ages of fifteen and forty.

IV. Etiology

A. It is a group of reactions (like schizophrenia in this respect).

B. It is usually considered a psychogenic (functional) psychosis, but like schizophrenia, the etiology is not definitely known.

C. Constitutional and hereditary factors

    1. The person with manic-depressive illness is commonly said to have the short and stout body type with rotund face (pyknic or endomorphic body build). Kretschmer reported a disproportionately large number of such body types among those with cyclothymic personalities and manic-depressive disease.

    2. The rhythmic nature of some cases often seems unrelated to any demonstrable psychological precipitating circumstances.

    3. Histories are said to reveal a high incidence of mental illness in the patient's families.

    4. A variety of possible factors has been named as of etiological importance, including dysfunction of the diencephalic centers involved in affective expression and the endocrine systems.

D. Genetic factors: The importance of genetic factors is not clear.

    1. Some authors believe the illness is genetically determined.

    2. Others say that the studies so far reported do not rule out educational transmission.

    3. Some reports indicate that manic-depressive illness is twenty-five times as frequent among the siblings of people who have the illness as among the general population.

    4. Other authorities say that if manic-depressive illness is found in one member of monozygotic twins, there is a 50 percent chance it will be found in the other.

    5. F. J. Kallmann's studies report 20 to 25 percent incidence in siblings of nonidentical twins and a 66 to 96 percent incidence in monozygotic twins.

E. Biological factors

    1. Neurophysiological, neurochemical, and neuropharmacological approaches have been opening up new avenues of understanding of behavior mechanisms. Recent research has been directed at steriod chemistry and catecholamine metabolism.

    2. There is a relative lack or absence of catecholamines in the brain of depressed persons.

    3. The spinal fluid seratonin levels are lower in depressed patients.

F. It is said to be much more frequent in the higher socioeconomic groups and among the professional class (manic-depressives are often successful).

G. Current theories regard psychogenic factors as the chief etiology. As one authority has said, even if constitutional factors are of importance, psychodynamic factors are rarely absent.

V. **Psychopathology**

A. Prepsychotic personality
1. Classically, the prepsychotic personality is cyclothymic (a personality characterized by alternating moods of sadness and elation with mood swings out of proportion to obvious stimuli).
2. Although not all have cyclothymic personality, most have prominent affective components in their personality makeup and many are described as extrovertive (i.e., their attention and energies are directed outwardly).
3. Some authors note obsessive-compulsive tendencies in the personalities of people who develop this reaction.

B. Precipitating factors may or may not be obvious in the individual attacks.

C. The social status of people with manic-depressive illness is well above that reported for schizophrenia and the organic brain syndromes.

D. The statements made about the psychopathology of depression in the section on depressive neurosis are generally applicable here, too. Others believe that the manic-depressive person has experienced a severe real, or fantasied loss at an early developmental stage. This is perceived as rejection which leads to the development of anger which becomes introjected and renders the person depressed.

E. The cyclic pattern of this illness has been related to alternating identification. During the depressive periods the patient identifies with the submissive mother-figure; in the manic phase he identifies with the over-aggressive paternal-figure.

F. The mood disturbances (elation or depression) may be considered to result from the manner in which the individual handles impulses, especially hostile and aggressive feelings.
1. If the restraint of one's censoring forces (conscience or superego) is removed, these impulses are freely expressed and elation (or mania) ensues.
2. If the censoring forces become reinforced, the impulses are directed against the individual (through the mechanism of

introjection) and deprcssion results. Here the effects are due to the rigid superego.

3. Thus, some have regarded manic-depressive illness as a "disease of the conscience."
4. Hostility can be said to be the common denominator in both depression and mania.

G. Manic behavior really represents massive denial of underlying depression. The person with elation may appear confident but is basically overdependent. When his dependency demands are unmet, hostility results which when repressed leads to depression.

VI. Symptomatology

A. Manic episode: In general, the manic episode is characterized by a flight of ideas, elated or grandiose mood, and psychomotor excitement (generalized physical and emotional overactivity). The individual with manic excitement seems to be running away from depression. Manic reactions are customarily divided into three degrees of disturbance: hypomania, acute mania, and delirious mania. These divisions are arbitrary and are made for the convenience of discussing the varying degrees of the disorder.

1. Hypomania
   a. Here the thought process rather than the thought content is disturbed. Each individual act seems normal, but when considered with other acts, the deviation becomes evident.
   b. The patient is active, ebullient, socially aggressive, talkative, boisterous, and flippant. He shows heightened emotional tone; he is effusive and euphoric. He is impatient and becomes irritable when he is frustrated. He is superficial and insensitive in his relationships with others. He is intolerant of criticism. He shows distractibility (responds quickly to stimuli, but his attention is not held) and loose association of speech (passes rapidly from topic to topic). He may be openly erotic in his speech or behavior.
   c. The patient remains oriented, lucid, and does not have delusions.
   d. The person who has chronic hypomania may accomplish much, although at times he may start many schemes which either fail or which he abandons.

e. He usually refuses to accept the fact that he is emotionally ill.

2. Acute mania

   a. Here the patient is obviously psychotic. He is loquacious, shows marked flight of ideas, and often exhibits incoherence of speech.

   b. He is extremely distractible, is often disoriented, and shows a tendency to rhyming, punning, and clang association (a play on words related by sound). Psychomotor excitement is marked. The patient shouts, throws things, and continually moves about. He is noisy, haughty, arrogant, and demanding. He is verbally abusive, expansive, overactive, and sometimes sexually indecent. At times he may become combative. Emotionally he shows aggression, irritability, and self-exaltation.

   c. Delusions of grandeur are often present (often in relationship to wealth, sexual prowess, or power). Hallucinations are also sometimes present.

   d. Paranoid traits are often evident.

3. Delirious mania (maniacal delirium): Marked aggravations of the conditions described under "Acute mania." Since the advent of modern psychiatric treatment, including the use of the somatic therapies and tranquilizers, the delirious manias are rarely seen.

B. Depressive episode: In general, the depressive episode is characterized by difficulty in thinking, depressive mood, and psychomotor retardation (a generalized diminution of emotional and physical responses). Depressive episodes are thought of as being divided into three degrees of disturbance: simple retardation, acute depression, and stuporous depression. These divisions are arbitrary and are made for convenience of discussion.

1. Simple retardation (mild depression)

   a. Such patients are only mildly ill.

   b. Movement and speech are slowed down. They may complain of ennui (a lack of interest or lassitude).

   c. Emotional depression is usually not marked and frequently is concealed from observers by the relatively normal facial expressions and relatively normal overt behavior of the patient. However, such individuals may complain of being lonely, sad, or pessimistic.

   d. They may complain of some appetite disturbance, sleep disturbance, and weight loss.

     e. Many complain of vague physical symptoms and may seek medical attention for these.

     f. Orientation is preserved.

  2. Acute depression: Here the depression is obvious.

     a. The patient is withdrawn. His speech is slow and often inaudible. Movements are obviously slowed down.

     b. Sometimes the patient shows agitation (motor restlessness, hand-wringing, pacing).

     c. Emotional depression is marked and obvious in the patient's behavior and facial expression. He speaks slowly and may even be mute or nearly so. Self-accusation and self-depreciation are prominent. He not only expresses the feeling of depression, but his appearance confirms this. His somatic symptoms are usually prominent and at times may become so fixed and bizarre that they become somatic delusions.

     d. Such patients are often suicidal risks. At times, they may even try to kill other people prior to taking their own lives. For example, a depressed mother may kill her child prior to making a suicidal attempt on her own life.

     e. Delusions and hallucinations are common.

  3. Stuporous depression (depressive stupor): This is the most severe degree of psychotic depression. The patient becomes mute, immobile, and severely regressed.

     a. Withdrawal is very marked in this type of depression.

     b. Such depressions are rarely seen since the advent of the somatic and the psychopharmacologic therapies.

VII. Clinical course

  A. The onset of this illness may be gradual or abrupt.

  B. The duration of untreated episodes varies from a few weeks to several years. In the past, the average untreated episode was about six months. Now, with modern hospitals and treatment techniques, the length of episodes can be reduced to a few weeks if the patient is treated promptly.

  C. The number of attacks is variable. An individual may have only one episode in a lifetime or may have numberless attacks. An individual may have alternating episodes of depression and elation, recurrent episodes of depression or elation only, etc. A common history is the occurrence of three to five episodes during a lifetime.

  D. Clinical subtypes:

    1. Manic-depressive illness, manic type (this disorder consists exclusively of manic episodes).

2. Manic-depressive illness, depressed type (this disorder consists exclusively of depressive episodes).
3. Manic-depressive illness, circular type (this disorder is distinguished by at least one attack of both a depressive episode and a manic episode).

VIII. Prognosis

A. Ordinarily the prognosis is good for the individual attack, but recurrence is fairly common.
B. The possible dangers of suicide should be kept in mind.
C. Deterioration of the personality between attacks usually does not occur. (This contrasts with what happens to personality between schizophrenic episodes.)
D. Psychopharmacologic and electroshock therapy have been of great value in shortening the duration of episodes but have probably not prevented recurrences (with the exception that patients who remain on maintenance therapy with tranquilizing or antidepressant drugs, or Lithium Carbonate may be able to remain free of attacks for long periods of time).

IX. Treatment

A. Hospitalization is usually indicated in most acute cases, although some of the milder depressive episodes can be treated outside of hospitals.
B. All manic episodes, even mild ones, should probably be treated in hospitals. Aside from the specific treatment for the episodes, the patient needs to be protected from the consequences and social embarrassment of his expansive behavior and poor judgment.
C. Tranquilizers (especially the phenothiazines, such as Chlorpromazine) and antidepressants (both the MAO inhibitor types, such as Tranylcypromine and the Iminodibenzyl Derivatives, such as Imipramine) have been beneficial in some of the milder reaction types.
D. Lithium carbonate will shorten periods of elation and may prevent attacks of either depression or elation when taken under a maintenance program.
E. Electroshock therapy accelerates the recovery of both depressive and manic episodes. In certain cases where the episodes have been frequent, EST has also been given on a "maintenance" basis to prevent relapses. Treatment is given at intervals of four, six, or eight weeks for several months or years. This has proved very effective in many cases of manic-depressive illness.

F. Psychotherapy during remission is sometimes thought to be helpful in preventing relapses. One difficulty here is that the patient often feels so well during remissions that he does not seek, or see the value of, treatment.

X. Case examples

A. Mr. S., a forty-one-year-old attorney, was admitted to the hospital in an acute manic episode. He was extremely hyperactive, distractible, irritable, and demanding. He showed a marked flight of ideas and expressed marked hostility toward his wife for what he described as infidelity. Eight years earlier, he developed a depressive episode following a severe infectious disease in his wife, and since that time he had developed manic symptoms every spring and depressive symptoms every fall. Prior to the onset of his illness, he was described as a perfectionistic, egotistical, and outgoing. Between episodes, he practiced law with above-average skill and showed no evidence of personality deterioration.

This is a classical case of manic-depressive illness. The patient's behavior on admission was typical of acute mania, showing elated mood, flight of ideas, and increased activity. Note also the absence of personality deterioration between attacks.

B. Mr. N., a fifty-five-year-old accountant, was admitted to the hospital with a severe depression which had begun following accidental injury of his son nine months earlier. He showed marked psychomotor retardation, refused to eat, and was mute most of the time. When he did speak, he expressed delusions of worthlessness, hopelessness, and nihilism. History from his family revealed that he had three previous episodes of depression, beginning at age twenty. Only the first attack had been severe enough to require hospital treatment. With the other episodes, he was able to function at his work, but with reduced efficiency. He was described as a quiet, shy, conscientious, sensitive person who worried unduly about his work and family.

This case is a manic-depressive illness characterized by several episodes of depression with absence of personality deterioration between attacks. This type was formerly classified as recurrent depression. The marked psychomotor retardation, the muteness, the refusal to eat, and delusions characterize the last attack as a stuporous depression.

C. John Ruskin (1819-1900) writer, critic, artist, and author of *Modern Painters* was the "archetype of manic-depressive, swing-

ing from elation to misery, always sensitive and always expressive."
D. Vincent W. Van Gogh (1853-1890), Dutch painter, suffered from mood swings, alternating between profound depression and extreme exuberance. On Christmas Eve, 1888, he cut off part of his left ear, and in July 1890, he committed suicide.

PSYCHOTIC-DEPRESSIVE REACTION

Synonym: reactive-depressive psychosis

   I. Definition: This diagnosis is reserved for those cases with a depressive mood attributable to some experience in which there is ordinarily no history of repeated depression or cyclothymic mood swings. In contrast to depressive neurosis, this condition is more severe and there is some impairment of reality testing.

  II. Occurrence: There are no reliable statistics on the existence of this condition.

 III. Etiology
   A. Genetic factors do not seem to be important in this reaction (contrast with manic-depressive illness).
   B. A number of factors have been suggested as being of etiological significance. Among these are:
   1. Environmental factors
   2. Various physical illnesses which make a person more vulnerable to emotional stress. This would include such things as infections or cardiac disease.
   3. Advanced age: Some writers feel that depression is more common in older people.
   4. Mutilating surgery: Depression may occur either as an anticipatory reaction or as a sequela.
   5. Grief: See discussion of grief at the beginning of this chapter.
   C. Perhaps the drug-induced depressions, such as those that have occurred with rauwolfia, can be classified here.

 IV. Clinical aspects
   A. The depression may vary in severity in individual cases.
   B. In general, the depressive symptoms are similar to those previously mentioned in this section and particularly resemble those of the depressive episode of a manic-depressive illness.

  V. Prognosis: The prognosis is very good.

VI. Treatment
A. Psychotherapy, of the supportive type, is often helpful. Environmental manipulation aids in the recovery.
B. Antidepressants (especially Iminodibenzyl derivatives, such as Imipramine and Amintriptyline) and tranquilizers (either the Phenothiazines such as Chlorpromazine or the minor tranquilizers such as Diazepam) are often useful.
C. Electroshock therapy shortens the course of the illness and is sometimes the only treatment that will relieve the depressive episode.
D. Hospitalization for treatment other than EST may be indicated.

REFERENCES

Ewalt, Jack R., and Farnsworth, Dana L. *Textbook of Psychiatry*. New York: McGraw-Hill Book Company, 1963, chap. VIII, XVIII, and XIX.

Freedman, Alfred M.; Kaplan, Harold I.; and Sadock, Benjamin J. *Modern Synopsis of Comprehensive Textbook of Modern Psychiatry*. Baltimore: The Williams & Wilkins Company, 1972, chap. XV, XVI, XIX, and XXVII.

Kolb, Larence C. *Modern Clinical Psychiatry*. 8th ed. Philadelphia: W. B. Saunders Company, 1973, chap. XXII and XXIV.

Involutional Melancholia

Synonyms: involutional psychotic reaction; involutional depression

I. **Definition:** Psychotic reaction with initial onset in the involutional period (late middle life). It is characterized most commonly by depressive affect, but occasionally by paranoid mentation.

II. **Introductory comments**
   A. Hippocrates described a condition of melancholia.
   B. Esquirol in the nineteenth century gave an accurate description of depressive reaction.
   C. Kraepelin distinguished the involutional depression from other types of depression in his classification in 1893, and first defined it as beginning in women after the menopause and during middle life in men.

III. **Occurrence**
   A. Three to five times more common among women.
   B. Occurs between ages forty and fifty-five in women; between ages fifty and sixty-five in men. Some studies indicate that the onset is most commonly three to seven years after menopause.
   C. It seems to occur more frequently in urban than in rural people and is thought to have a higher incidence among the lower socioeconomic group, the divorced, and the widowed.

D. "Involutional thinking" (introspective ruminations about the past and the future): Occurs in the above age groups and is an important dynamic consideration in the adjustment that people make to the climacterium (involutional period).

IV. Etiology

A. In the past, some authors have stressed the importance of changes in the endocrine and reproductive systems which occur at the climacterium. (However, it should be noted that hormonal replacement therapy has been largely unsuccessful in treating involutional reaction.)

B. Most authorities now regard these disorders as primarily psychological reactions to the climacterium (or the psychological implications of the physiological changes incident to the climacterium).

V. Psychopathology

A. Prepsychotic personality

1. Most commonly the person who develops involutional melancholia has an obsessive-compulsive personality: rigid, inflexible, superego-dominated (meticulous, worrisome, thrifty, intolerant, stubborn, scrupulously honest, and restricted in interests).

   a. Such traits make an individual inflexible and thus limit his adaptability and methods of self-expression.

   b. As a consequence, the stress of the involutional period is more difficult.

2. The second most common type of prepsychotic personality is the passive-aggressive personality. Such a person shows both passivity and aggressiveness. The aggressiveness may be expressed in passive ways.

B. At the climacterium, most people have reached their peak of achievement. Thus, there may be nothing to look forward to. In addition, in the United States culture, emphasis and value have been placed on youth—rather than maturity.

C. The death of a loved-one (spouse, relative, or close friend) may be of dynamic significance in some cases. This is especially true if there is an attendant loss of dependency gratification.

D. In women

1. The involutional period has many cultural implications which may be disturbing. Included are the loss of physical attractiveness, the threatened loss of personal warmth and sexual desirability.

2. Loneliness may be an important factor.

3. Nonacceptance of aging is sometimes of importance.
4. For those who have been compulsively devoted to their families, the departure of children from the home to college, employment, or marriage removes the chief source of sublimation and leaves them with an emotional void.
5. Even the presence of a retired husband in the home may disturb her compulsive routines.
6. Some authorities have regarded involutional reaction as a regressive process in which there is a reenactment of the conflict of the small girl.

E. In men
1. Waning sexual potency and reduction of competitive productivity are factors often to be considered etiologically significant. These may be equated with the loss of masculinity.
2. The reaction often seems closely related to retirement from active work, especially if the man has no interests or activities to substitute.

F. Psychoanalytically, involutional melancholia is regarded as the individual's reaction of grief and anger to a real or imagined loss in later life.

G. Occasionally, physical trauma, mutilating surgery, or some physical illness may initiate the onset of this disorder.

H. In general, the person of rigid character (anal-sadistic) seems especially susceptible to frustrations during the involutional period.

VI. Clinical types
A. Involutional melancholia (involutional depressive reaction) is the most frequent type.
B. Involutional paranoid state (involutional paraphrenia)
1. This psychosis is classified under paranoid states in the new nomenclature but is discussed here.
2. It is a paranoid psychosis with initial onset of delusion formation in the involution period.

VII. Symptoms: Most of these reactions are depressive in nature. A few are of the paranoid type.
A. Involutional melancholia
1. The classical involutional melancholia is an agitated depression. However, cases vary from mild retardations to severe delusional depressions. Delusions may be somatic (concerning the body or bodily functions) or nihilistic (delusions of nonexistence of the self or part of the self).
2. Self-depreciation: This may vary from feelings of inade-

quacy with indecisiveness to delusional self-accusation and suicidal preoccupation.
3. Agitation: Varies from mild restlessness to extreme psychomotor expression of emotional tension. Sometimes there is a rather prolonged prodromal period of anxiety and apprehension. Agitation is not always present.
4. Somatic symptoms: Some somatic complaint is usually present, and oftentimes it is this which first prompts the patient to seek medical attention. As a matter of fact, the appearance of the depressive state is often preceded by a period of hypochondriacal preoccupation. Such symptoms can be found in any body system. Commonly, these are gastrointestinal or cardiovascular. In severe cases, the somatic symptoms may be so fixed that they are really somatic delusions.
5. Often the history indicates some overt situational change which precedes or initiates the illness—for example, retirement from work; marriage of children; relocation in a new home.
6. In women, the onset is usually not too closely associated with the cessation of menses (menopause), but antedates or postdates this.
7. The initial attack occurs in women between forty and fifty-five and in men between fifty and sixty-five.

B. Involutional paranoid state:
1. A reaction characterized chiefly by paranoid delusions.
2. It is similar to other paranoid disorders except the onset is in the involutional age period.
3. The prognosis for this type is somewhat less favorable than for the melancholic type.
4. Paranoid features may also be present in the involutional depressive reactions (and vice versa).
5. The prepsychotic personality of this type of individual shows paranoid traits and tendency to project in addition to compulsive characteristics.

VIII. Prognosis
A. If untreated, the prognosis for people with involutional reactions is very poor. Many would not recover or would improve only after many months or years of illness.
B. With the advent of somatic treatment, the recovery rate has been excellent (80 percent to 90 percent).
C. Prognosis is better in the younger, more intelligent patient. Prognosis is also better when treatment is instituted early and when there has been an acute onset of severe symptomatology.

    D. A history of previous good adjustment, adequate ego-strength, and a favorable post-treatment environment are also hopeful factors.

    E. Factors which suggest a poor prognosis:
      1. The presence of organic brain damage.
      2. The presence of marked paranoid or schizoid features.

IX. Treatment

    A. Electroshock therapy is often the treatment of choice and has largely been responsible for the favorable outlook in these disorders.

    B. Antidepressant and tranquilizer medications are often useful in the milder forms and sometimes are used as adjuncts to electroshock therapy also.

    C. Follow-up individual psychotherapy is often helpful to permit the patient to gain insight into dynamics and to prevent relapses. However, long-term intensive psychotherapy is usually not indicated.

    D. In rare instances, prefrontal lobotomy has been recommended for severe crippling agitation and depression that is rarely seen in this condition.

X. Case example: Mr. J., a sixty-five-year-old man, was admitted to the hospital complaining of loss of appetite, insomnia, weight loss, depression, and constipation. His illness began six months earlier when he was retired from his job as a shop foreman. He had always enjoyed good physical health and never had emotional illness previously. He had no interests aside from his work and was described by his family as serious, conscientious, rigid, and hard-working. On admission he was obviously depressed and cried frequently. He showed psychomotor retardation, complained of difficulty in thinking, and was preoccupied with his symptom of constipation, believing that his bowels had dried up because he had no bowel movements. He was self-deprecatory and at times did not wish to eat because he thought he was unworthy. He made an excellent recovery with ECT and has remained well for several years.

The onset of a delusional depression in the involutional period characterizes this as an involutional depressive reaction. Note also that the illness began when he was retired. The absence of agitation is atypical. Often, however, agitation does not develop until after the patient has had the illness for several months.

REFERENCES

Freedman, Alfred M.; Kaplan, Harold I.; and Sadock, Benjamin J. *Modern Synopsis of Comprehensive Textbook of Modern Psychiatry.* Baltimore: The William & Wilkins Company, 1972, chap. XV.

Kolb, Lawrence C. *Modern Clinical Psychiatry.* 8th ed. Philadelphia: W. B. Saunders Company, 1973, chap. XXII.

"My mind is troubled, like a fountain
stirr'd
and I myself see not the bottom of it."

**Shakespeare: TROILUS AND
CRESSIDA**

Schizophrenia

I. **Historical notes**
   A. The syndromes that are now classified under schizophrenia have been recognized for a long time, although in the past they have carried varying diagnoses.
   B. B. A. Morel (1860) introduced the term *demence precoce* to describe psychosis in a fourteen-year-old boy.
   C. E. Hecker (1871) described hebephrenia as a progressive psychotic illness of rapid onset beginning in adolescence.
   D. K. Kahlbaum (1874) described catatonia, or "tension insanity," and assumed it to be a symptom of some organic brain disease. His description was of a condition characterized by muteness, immobility, waxy flexibility, etc.
   E. Emil Kraepelin (1896), believing that all of the above syndromes were related, classified them into one group called dementia praecox.
   F. Adolph Meyer (1906) introduced the concept of dementia praecox as a reaction type (parergastic reaction).
   G. Eugen Bleuler (1911) coined the term *schizophrenia* to emphasize the "splitting" of the personality (from the Greek: *schizo*—"to split"; *phren*—"mind").

II. **Definition:** A group of disorders manifested by characteristic disturbances of thinking, mood, and behavior. Disturbances in thinking are marked by alterations of concept formation which may lead to misinterpretation of reality and sometimes to delusions and hallucinations which frequently appear psychologically self-protective. Corollary mood changes include ambivalent, constricted, and inappropriate emotional responsiveness and loss of empathy with others. Behavior may be withdrawn, regressive, and bizarre (DSM-II, 1968).

III. Incidence
A. About 1 percent of the population.
B. About 25 percent of all psychotic disorders but 50 percent to 60 percent of the population of state hospitals.
C. Twenty-five percent of *all* hospital beds in the United States are occupied by schizophrenics.
D. There are an estimated 320,000 hospitalized schizophrenics in the United States.
E. It seems probable that there are as many schizophrenics outside of hospitals as are inside of them. Such persons are sometimes referred to as ambulatory schizophrenics.

IV. Age of onset
A. Although schizophrenia may begin at almost any age, it is primarily a disease of younger age groups and the onset usually occurs somewhere from late childhood to middle life. Some cases have been reported in early childhood (see "Childhood Schizophrenia").
B. Most frequently begins in adolescence or early adult life.
C. It is not as rare in childhood as was once believed.

V. Etiology
A. The cause of schizophrenia is unknown. Since this is probably a group of reactions, it is quite unlikely that a single cause will ever be found.
B. Theories of etiology can be divided into:
   1. Psychological
   2. Sociocultural
   3. Organic
C. Genetic factors
   1. Some studies do suggest the operation of a genetic factor in schizophrenic disorders. However, most authorities who believe there is some genetic determination also think that other subsequent factors (biological, psychological, or so-

cial) are necessary for the production of a schizophrenic disorder.

2. Studies indicate that children of schizophrenic parents are much more likely to develop the disorder than the general population (expectancy in children of one schizophrenic parent is 16 percent versus 0.85 percent for the general population. In families where both parents are schizophrenic, the expectancy in the children is 40 percent).

3. Twin studies (F. J. Kallmann) suggest a genetic factor.
   a. Monozygotic (identical) twins: If present in one twin, in 85 percent or more in the cases it is also found in the other twin.
   b. Dizygotic (fraternal) twins: If present in one twin, in only 14 percent of the cases is it found in the other twin (approximately the same expectancy as in full siblings).
   c. The presence of a genetic factor does not necessarily invalidate a psychogenic etiology.

4. The significance of genetic factors is questioned by many authorities because statistical studies have not taken into account early environmental forces (especially intrafamily relationships).

D. Organic factors
1. Asthenic body build was thought to be more commonly affected, but this is certainly not true in all instances.
2. Many organic, particularly physiological, changes have been reported. Some of these have been incidental findings not specifically related to schizophrenic reactions, and others, though apparently related to the disorder, may be secondary rather than primary.
3. Earlier neuropathological studies suggested differences in the brains of schizophrenics as compared to normals. However, recent studies do not confirm this and currently the opinion is that the brains of schizophrenics are no different than those of normal people on neuropathological examination.
4. Recent research has been aimed at endocrinological studies, especially steroid chemistry and catechol amine metabolism. Some authorities have reported "abnormal" compounds in the blood of schizophrenics, but the significance of these is not known.
5. At the present time, the organic findings do not permit any definite theoretical conclusions.

E. Psychological theories
   1. Current theories seem more concerned with the possible psychogenic etiology of the schizophrenic reactions.
   2. Although it is found in every culture and in all socio-economic groups, its greatest incidence is in the lower socioeconomic group.
   3. There are those who regard it as a social disorder rather than a psychiatric illness.

VI. **Conceptions of schizophrenia**
   A. Emil Kraepelin: Dementia praecox resulted from injury to the germ plasm or from some metabolic disorder which caused autointoxication. He was the first to include hebephrenic, catatonic, and paranoid type reactions under the one syndrome.
   B. Eugen Bleuler: His concept was wider than Kraepelin's, and although he believed this illness to be primarily of physical origin, he did consider certain secondary symptoms (such as delusions, hallucinations, and mannerisms) to be of psychogenic origin. He emphasized the "splitting of the various mental functions" (i.e., the coexistence of disharmonious complexes). He regarded the formal mechanism underlying schizophrenic symptoms as the loosening of association (e.g., in blocking).
   C. Adolph Meyer: Regarded this as a maladaptation reaction ("The accumulation of lifelong faulty habits of adaptation in the setting of an inferior, psychobiological endowment.") He emphasized the longitudinal (versus the cross-sectional) psychological factors.
   D. Sigmund Freud: Regarded this as withdrawal and regression associated with a weak ego. There is a return to early narcissism, that is, the libido is withdrawn from external objects and directed toward the ego.
   E. Carl Jung: The psyche is unable to rid itself of a complex and can no longer adapt to the surroundings; thus separation from reality results. He thought that delusions, hallucinations, and other schizophrenic symptoms were due to an autochthonous complex—that is, a group of ideas which, because they were disturbing, were removed from consciousness and maintained in an independent existence.
   F. Harry Stack Sullivan: Regarded schizophrenia as the indirect outcome of unhealthy, interpersonal relationships between the child (who later becomes schizophrenic) and the parent.

G. The double-bind theory: In 1960, Bateson suggested a theory of schizophrenia in which he hypothesized that learning occurs in a context with formal characteristics; also, the context is regarded as occurring within a broader context ("metacontext"). Occurrences in the narrow context will be affected by the metacontext. There may be conflict or discordance between the metacontext and the context. Conditioned learning in the context set in a metacontext which is punitive toward such learning would produce discordance. Thus the individual is confronted with the dilemma of "being wrong in the primary context or being right for the wrong reasons or in a wrong way. This is the so-called double bind." Whether such a double bind is unique to schizophrenic patients is not really known at this time.

According to Noyes and Kolb, "the schizophrenic may be seen as fixed in an intense, emotional relationship with a parent who, by the contradictions between her verbal remarks and behavior, makes it impossible for the former to discriminate properly or to respond for clarification, as his questioning is treated as a threat to the needed relationship by the parent. A concrete example is a schizophrenic adolescent who, tied to his mother verbally, is encouraged to use initiative in his schoolwork, yet when he attempts to leave home to visit the library, he is told he must not do so as the parent needs him and will become ill in his absence. Such a double bind restricts and confuses the development of clear communications, since the parent's position is inconsistent and also limits the son's healthful socialization with others, from which he might learn progressive social discriminations and develop the potentiality for evolving other healthy relations. Whether the double bind is characteristic of schizophrenic families alone or has special features for such families is not known."*

H. Silvano Arieti: Regards schizophrenia as a reaction to an extremely severe state of anxiety originating in childhood and reactivated later in life. It occurs when no other possibility of adjustment is available to the patient.

I. Family psychopathology: The studies in this area have been made from two points of view:

1. Studies concerned with psychodynamic interaction between individuals.

2. Socially-oriented studies which seem concerned with the

*From A. P. Noyes, and L. C. Kolb, *Modern Clinical Psychiatry,* 7th ed., (Philadelphia: W. B. Saunders Company, 1968).

individual's reaction to psychopathology within the family constellation. Most of the studies have been concerned with psychopathology in the parental family, although some have been concerned with the psychopathology in the marital family.

J. Phenomenological-existential concepts: Binswanger is the best-known exponent. His case reports concern themselves with the underlying structure that existed prior to the illness, etc.

VII. Psychopathology

A. Clinically, most psychiatrists regard schizophrenic reaction as regression. (See Freudian concept, previously mentioned, and regression under "Adjustive Patterns.")

1. There is withdrawal of interest from the environment and loss of interest in object relationships.

2. According to psychoanalytic theory, this regression is to a level at which the schizophrenic, like the infant, is incapable of distinguishing himself from his environment (regression to primary narcissism).

B. Those having paranoid delusions are also overusing the mechanism of projection (see "Adjustive Patterns").

C. The prepsychotic personality is often schizoid (introvert).

D. Precipitating factors may or may not be evident and vary with the individual's vulnerability.

1. May be somatic, such as pregnancy ("postpartum psychosis") or a physical illness.

2. May be emotional, such as marital difficulty, an unhappy love affair or, at times, even trivial emotional interactions.

3. The onset may be gradual with no obvious precipitating factors.

VIII. Symptomatology

A. Since our present-day concept of this disorder actually includes varying clinical pictures, it is difficult to present a "typical" cluster of symptoms which are characteristic of all cases.

B. The symptomatology most commonly associated with this reaction can be conveniently discussed under the following headings:

1. Thinking disturbances:

a. The disturbance of thinking is the most characteristic aspect of this disorder. The schizophrenic thinks in a concrete rather than a conceptual way with loss of abstract attitude.

    b. There are delusions. These are most commonly persecutory, but may be grandiose or somatic.

    c. Ideas of reference, influence, or suspiciousness may also be present.

    d. The stream of thought may show vagueness, circumstantiality, or neologisms.

    e. Often shows blocking.

2. Perceptual disturbances: Hallucinations may be present. These are less frequent than delusions, and when present are most commonly auditory.

3. Emotional disturbances

    a. Emotional response is generally reduced.

    b. Emotional response is often inadequate.

    c. Emotional response may be inappropriate with the patient showing unexpected, silly, or bizarre reactions.

    d. Some appear to be tense. This is usually found in the acute phase.

    e. Abnormal emotions such as states of exaltation, feelings of omnipotence, and religious ecstasies may be evident.

4. Behavior disturbances: May vary from mild, withdrawal, all the way to severe, bizzare changes. Included are mannerisms, negativism, stereotypy, echopraxia, catatonic stupor or excitement, automatic obedience.

5. Verbal disturbances: Verbal productions may vary from incoherence all the way to severe mutism. Included are incoherence, neologisms, verbigeration, stilted language, excessive concretions, and symbolism.

6. Somatic symptoms: No specific physical symptoms are associated with schizophrenia. Often, however, the early schizophrenic complains of multiple physical symptoms. Sometimes these have a hypochondriacal or neurasthenic quality.

C. Of all these symptoms, the inappropriateness or inadequacy of emotional response is the most characteristic.

IX. Clinical types: Because of the varied clinical picture, cases are classified into different clinical types depending upon the predominant symptomatology.

A. Simple type

1. The chief characteristics are emotional blunting, apathy, and preoccupation with fantasy life. Sometimes appears intellectually dull. There are no delusions or hallucinations.

2. Often there is a long history of inadequate social adjustment and inability to relate well to others. Thus, the onset is often gradual and insidious but is usually manifested in adolescence or early adult life. The point at which a schizoid personality becomes schizophrenic is oftentimes arbitrary.

3. Prognosis: The prognosis for recovery is usually hopeless, although the process of schizophrenic deterioration sometimes reaches a "plateau" of arrested progress and the individual may continue to function at a borderline or marginal level.

4. Case example: Betty, an eighteen-year-old college freshman, was brought to the hospital by her mother. She had always been a shy girl whose quiet, conforming behavior was regarded as seriousness or studiousness. About one year earlier, the mother noted that Betty began to show progressive loss of interest in her associates and her schoolwork and seemed to prefer being by herself. Shortly after she entered college, this withdrawal became more evident and, in addition, she complained of dizziness, nausea, and vomiting. Examination by the school physician had failed to reveal any physical explanation for her symptoms.

   In the ward she showed unusual and, at times, regressive behavior. She would lie in bed with the covers drawn over her head, refusing to look at the examiner and answering questions only by nodding or shaking her head. Her attitude was frequently one of uncooperation with childlike bursts of irritability. On occasions, however, she was listless and uncommunicative.

5. In the preceding case can be noted the previous schizoid personality, a gradual onset but with definite schizophrenic manifestations in late adolescence. Her behavior was characterized by inappropriateness, apathy, regression, and absence of delusions and hallucinations. Oftentimes such patients have some accompanying somatic symptoms.

B. Hebephrenic type (from Hebe, the goddess of youth)

1. Chief characteristics: There is marked regression to primitive, unorganized, and uninhibited behavior. Onset in adolescence. Symptoms are bizarre. There is obvious emotional disturbance with marked inappropriateness of affect, extremely poor contact with reality, dilapidated appearance, fantastic delusions and hallucinations. Grinning

and grimacing are often present. Sometimes there are outbursts of laughing. The behavior can best be described as silly.

2. Often the prepsychotic personality is schizoid but the onset of psychotic symptoms is more definite than in the simple type.

3. Prognosis: Many show progressive deterioration.

4. Case example: Mary, a twenty-one-year-old stenographer, was brought to the hospital by the police who had been called after she had entered a strange residence at 1:00 a.m. because of an uncontrollable urge to urinate. She had always been a shy, introverted, and intensely religious girl. Three years earlier after high school graduation she had a "nervous breakdown" which required six months hospitalization. She showed improvement following treatment but still seemed shy, self-contained, and at times inappropriate in her behavior. Three days before admission she became restless, sleepless, and spent the night on her knees in continuous prayer. The following morning she seemed elated and became upset by several minor, commonplace incidents. She started out for work but in response to "voices" went instead to religious services at a nearby church. The second night was likewise spent in continuous prayer. The following morning she again started out for work but became confused and returned home. The evening preceding admission she boarded a bus to attend church but became confused "because my friend Anne prayed that I would get mixed up" and left the bus far from church. She wandered about aimlessly, finally entering the strange residence at 1:00 a.m.

On admission she was obviously disturbed. She was preoccupied with religious and moral ideas and said that God was talking to her through the newspapers, radio, and television. She repeatedly misidentified the ward personnel as apostles, disciples, and other biblical characters. Her affect was euphoric and inappropriate. She showed increased motor activity, making frequent changes in posture and moving about the room aimlessly. She was unkempt and continuously disrobed.

Despite a three-month stay in the hospital during which time she received thirty electroconvulsive treatments, she did not show any sustained improvement in her behavior

and she was committed to a state hospital for prolonged
care.
5. In this case can be noted the schizoid prepsychotic personality, the rather definite onset of psychotic symptoms in
   adolescence, the obvious emotional disturbance at the time
   of admission, and the bizzare nature of her symptoms.
   Note also the bizarre delusions and hallucinations.
C. Paranoid type
   1. Chief characteristics: Paranoid delusions that are "illogical"
      and unsystematized are the most prominent feature. These
      are usually of a persecutory nature, but may be grandiose.
      The patient often does not react appropriately to his delu-
      sions. He is often reserved, guarded, and suspicious in his
      behavior and sometimes hostile.
   2. Onset often abrupt and is usually in adult life.
   3. Prognosis: Usually good for a given episode but recur-
      rences are fairly common. With the neuroleptic drugs and
      EST, the prognosis has been markedly improved.
   4. Case example: Mrs. L., a thirty-year-old housewife, was
      brought to the hospital by her family because she had
      exhibited strange behavior for the preceding seven
      months. This was characterized by withdrawal, inappro-
      priate mood, preoccupation with religious ideas, and delu-
      sions that her husband and the family physician were "try-
      ing to poison the food." In preschool years she had been
      overly attached to her mother but subsequently became so
      interested in outdoor activities that she was considered a
      "tomboy."
      In the hospital she was markedly suspicious of the entire
      staff, accusing them of poisoning her food, talking about
      her, gambling, etc. She said she received messages from
      Christ whose voice came to her over the radio. Much of the
      time she was withdrawn but at times talked readily—
      though inappropriately. Her affect was flattened.
      Following a course of electroconvulsive therapy she
      showed good improvement and returned home. Eighteen
      months later the same symptoms recurred and she was
      readmitted to the hospital. Though the second episode was
      more refractory to treatment, she did improve sufficiently
      to return home after eight months.
   5. In this case the features which classify it as paranoid
      schizophrenia are the prominent paranoid delusions and

hallucinations, the inappropriate behavior and flattening of affect. Note also the onset in early adult life and the good response to treatment of the first episode.

D. Catatonic type

1. Catatonic stupor (withdrawal): This is characterized by mutism, negativism, stereotypies, echopraxia, mannerisms, posturizing, waxy flexibility, automatic obedience, retention of excretions, and refusal to eat.

2. Catatonic excitement: This is characterized by extreme psychomotor agitation. The patient becomes violently excited, destructive, and assaultive. He talks continuously and his stream of speech is incoherent. Such a patient seems motivated from within and is always dangerous.

3. Onset of both is usually sudden and the course is usually short.

4. Prognosis: good for recovery from the episode but guarded for future recurrences.

5. Case example of catatonic stupor: Miss J., a thirty-nine-year-old secretary, was brought to the hospital by her two sisters because she exhibited bizarre behavior for the preceding week. She was described as a quiet, reserved person who had few friends and preferred to remain by herself. Although she danced occasionally, she was generally shy in the company of men. She showed no symptoms of emotional illness until seven days earlier when she suddenly began to abstain from food. Five days later she expressed religious delusions, became self-condemnatory, refused to go to bed at night, and demanded to see a priest at 3:00 A.M. A few hours later she was admitted to a general hospital and received intravenous feedings because of her refusal to eat. She would not remain in bed and left the hospital against advice. At home she continued to refuse food and her sisters sought her admission to the hospital.

On admission she was negativistic, refusing food, medication, and nursing care. She was mute most of the time, and when she did speak she expressed religious delusions and hallucinations. She showed posturizing, that is, assumed uncomfortable postures for long periods, and exhibited waxy flexibility, that is, her extremities would remain in positions in which they were placed.

She recovered from this episode after a course of electroconvulsive therapy and was discharged to her home at the end of one month. A few weeks later she had a recurrence of symptoms. This second episode also responded rather promptly to treatment and she was discharged after six weeks. She has remained well for several years.

The characteristic features in the foregoing case of catatonic stupor are the sudden onset of negativism, mutism, posturizing, and waxy flexibility; the good response to treatment in both instances; the prepsychotic schizoid personality.

6. Case example of catatonic excitement: P. H., a twenty-year-old college student, was brought to the hospital in restraints by the police. His illness had become manifest one day prior to admission when he began expressing delusions of grandeur and persecution. He left his fraternity house without telling anyone where he was going and remained away all night. About two hours before admission, the police were summoned to pick him up in a nearby suburb because of bizarre behavior characterized by agitation, assaultiveness, and disrobing. Before the onset of his illness he was described as conscientious, compulsive, and meek. He resisted accepting responsibility and had an "inferiority complex."

On admission he was uncooperative, mute, belligerant, agitated, and assaultive. He refused food, medications, and nursing care and was careless of his excreta. After a series of electroconvulsive treatments he became cooperative and calm. Treatment was continued in another hospital where he was transferred in order to be nearer his parental home.

In this case, the mutism, negativism, agitation, assaultiveness, and violent behavior characterize this as catatonic excitement.

E. Periodic catatonia: This is a rare form of episodic catatonia which is related to shifts in the individual's metabolic nitrogen balance. Maintenance on neuroleptic drugs prevents recurrence.

F. Acute schizophrenic episode
   1. Cases included under this diagnosis are those with an acute onset of schizophrenic symptoms often associated with confusion, emotional turmoil, perplexity, ideas of reference, dissociative phenomena, excitement, depression, or fear.
   2. The onset is acute and is often accompanied by a pronounced affective coloring of either elation or depression.

3. In time, these patients may take on the characteristics of catatonic, hebephrenic, or paranoid schizophrenia.
4. In many cases, the patient recovers within a few weeks, but sometimes his disorganization becomes progressive.

G. Chronic undifferentiated type: This category is for patients who show mixed schizophrenic symptomatology and who demonstrate definite schizophrenic thought, affect, and behavior, but who are not classifiable under the other types.

H. Schizophrenia, latent type
1. This category is for patients having clear symptoms of schizophrenia, but no history of a psychotic schizophrenic episode.
2. Disorders previously diagnosed as incipient, pseudo-neurotic, pseudopsychopathic, or borderline schizophrenia are categorized here.
3. In this form of schizophrenia, the underlying psychotic process is often masked by complaints which are ordinarily regarded as neurotic.
4. The diagnosis rests on the constellative evaluation of a group of symptoms, even though in any given case it is not necessary to have all the symptoms present.
5. Symptoms
   a. Autistic (self-centered) and dereistic (abstract or unreal) life approach.
   b. Withdrawal from reality (less than in classical schizophrenia).
   c. Widespread and diffuse ambivalence (really, polyvalence).
   d. No gross affective changes.
   e. Pan-anxiety (all-pervading and overwhelming).
   f. Pan-neurosis (many symptoms, such as anxiety, phobias, obsessions, depressions, as well as somatic symptoms).
   g. No gross thinking disorders, but minor ones evident on psychometric testing.
   h. Vagueness of elaboration on symptoms and inability to associate freely (indistinct in describing symptoms).
   i. Occasional micropsychotic episodes (symptoms mild and of short duration). Three elements are usually present:
      (1) Hypochondriacal symptoms
      (2) Ideas of reference
      (3) Depersonalization (feelings of strangeness or unreality about self or environment)

6. Course: protracted and of long duration.
I. Schizophrenia, residual type
This term is for patients who show signs of schizophrenia following a psychotic schizophrenic episode.

X. Childhood schizophrenia
A. Definition: This category is for cases in which the symptoms appear before puberty. The disorder may be manifested by autistic, atypical, and withdrawn behavior; failure to develop identity separate from the mothers' and general unevenness, gross immaturity, and inadequacy in development. (DSM-II)
B. Most of these patients have disturbed body image.
C. Until relatively recently many believed that schizophrenia did not occur before puberty. In the past several years, cases of childhood schizophrenia have been reported with increasing frequency in the literature, though there still seems to be some controversy whether such cases are really the same as schizophrenia in adults. Some believe childhood schizophrenia is a different disorder than adult schizophrenia and refer to such disorders as "atypical children." While there is controversy about the etiology, there is an increasing trend to regard the illness as the result of an interaction of constitutional and psychogenic factors.
D. In 1943, Kanner first reported a psychotic reaction occurring in children under the age of two years which he labeled "early infantile autism." This was characterized by profound withdrawal, obsessive desire to preserve sameness, and mutism. According to Kanner, this reaction is indistinguishable from childhood schizophrenia. The parents of these youngsters were said to be "sophisticated" but lacked warmth in their relationships with their children.
E. A reaction similar to infantile autism but first manifest after the second year has been called symbiotic infantile psychosis. The chief difference from infantile autism is that it occurs in youngsters whose emotional development seemed relatively normal for the first few years of life.
F. The clinical picture may differ from schizophrenic reactions occurring in other age groups because of the immaturity of the person at the time of the onset.

XI. Course
A. Formerly regarded as a progressive disorder with a poor, or hopeless, prognosis.

B. Currently, psychiatrists are much more optimistic about arrest and recovery in this illness, chiefly because of the favorable effects of the somatic therapies and psychotropic drugs.

C. As can be noted from the classification, episodic types of schizophrenia are now recognized. These are oftentimes followed by symptom-free periods. Occasionally, individuals have been observed to have a single, mild schizophrenic (or schizophrenic-like) attack without having any recurrences.

D. Because clinically schizophrenia occurs either in "attacks" or as a progressive disease, some psychiatrists speak of "reactive" and "process" schizophrenia.

XII. **Prognosis:** In general, the prognosis is guarded. Certain criteria have become more or less accepted for prognosticating the outcome of any case of schizophrenia.

A. The following are considered favorable prognostic signs:
1. Sudden onset
2. Conspicuous precipitating factors
3. Catatonic symptoms
4. The presence of affective symptoms (depression or elation)
5. The presence of confusion
6. History of good previous social adjustment
7. If symptoms have been present for less than one year
8. Married patients have a better outlook than single, divorced, or widowed persons
9. If the individual has a job to which he can return
10. If he is cooperative in the treatment regime

B. The following are considered unfavorable signs:
1. History of previous attacks
2. Schizoid prepsychotic personality
3. Absence of conspicuous precipitating factors
4. Family history of mental illness
5. If onset is before adolescence or after age forty
6. If symptoms have been present for more than one year

XIII. **Treatment**

A. The type of treatment depends upon the type and severity of the disorder.

B. Since the etiology is incompletely understood, the treatment has largely been empirical. Treatment can be divided into:
1. Psychological
2. Somatic (organic)

C. Psychological treatment: Psychotherapy is sometimes helpful in the early stages and is often used in recovered patients as a prophylactic measure.

D. Although some schizophrenics can make a marginal adjustment extramurally, hospitalization is frequently indicated in most cases, at least for some period of time. So-called "total push" therapy (Myerson) is often of value in chronic, deteriorated cases.

E. One or more of the somatic therapies is often necessary.
   1. Electroshock therapy (EST) is used in acute cases.
   2. Regressive electroshock therapy (REST) or intensive electroshock therapy is sometimes used in chronic, relapsing, or latent forms.
   3. Insulin coma therapy has been used in severe chronic types. This type of treatment is rarely used now.
   4. Prefrontal lobotomy may be used occasionally for certain chronic or relapsing cases which have responded inadequately, or only temporarily, to electroshock therapy or insulin coma therapy.

F. Tranquilizing drugs:
   1. Since their first appearance in the United States in 1954, tranquilizers have been used extensively in the treatment of schizophrenia.
   2. The tranquilizing drugs most useful in schizophrenia are the phenothiazine group: This includes chlorpromazine (Thorazine), triflouperazine (Stelazine), perphenazine (Trilafon), thioridazine (Mellaril), and fluphenazine (Prolixin, Permitil).

G. Commonly, the most effective treatment program is one combining somatic, psychological, and environmental approaches.

REFERENCES

Bateson, Gregory. "Minimal Requirements for a Theory of Schizophrenia." American Medical Association. *Archives of General Psychiatry,* 2(1960): 477.

Bellek, L. *Dementia Praecox.* New York: Grune & Stratton, Inc., 1949.

Bosselman, B. C. *Neurosis and Psychosis.* 3rd. ed. Springfield, Illinois: Charles C. Thomas Publishers, 1964.

Freedman, Alfred M.; Kaplan, Harold I.; and Sadock, Benjamin J. *Modern Synopsis of Comprehensive Textbook of Modern Psychiatry.* Baltimore: The William & Wilkins Company, 1972.

Kanner, L. "Problems of Nosology and Psychodynamics of Early Infantile Autism." *Am. Journ. Orthopsychiat.* 19 (July, 1949): 416.

Kolb, Lawrence C. *Modern Clinical Psychiatry.* 8th ed. Philadelphia: W. B. Saunders Company, 1973.

Paranoid States

I. **Definition:** Psychotic disorders in which a delusion, generally per-
    secutory or gandiose, is the essential abnormality (DSM-II). They
    are usually without hallucinations or schizophrenic behavior.

II. **Introduction**
    A. All of these syndromes are characterized by overuse of the
        mechanism of projection (see chapter on "Adjustive Pat-
        terns").
    B. Although overuse of projection is pathological, it is a defense
        mechanism that is fairly commonly employed. For example,
        blaming others for our own mistakes; blaming social ills on
        minority groups; often certain militant groups such as an-
        tivivisectionists and antiflouridationists may be overusing the
        mechanism of projection; most all of us are usually critical of
        our own shortcomings when we find them in others.
    C. People with paranoid conditions show hyperalertness, over-
        suspiciousness, reality distortion, and delusions.
    D. The delusions can be:
        1. Jealous: The jealousy is usually more persistent and pro-
            found than normal jealousy. There is usually some grain of
            truth in the pathological jealousy but the constructs on
            which it rests are based on inadequate evidence. In the

Shakespearean drama, Othello becomes furiously jealous of his innocent wife and his loyal lieutenant, Michael Cassio. He executes his wife with his own hands. After killing her, he learns of her innocence and he judges and executes himself.

2. Erotic: These delusions may concern infidelity, sexual exploitation, change of sex, or the grandiose idea of being loved by someone else, often a famous person (who must keep secret the love relationship).

3. Grandiose (exalted): Delusions of having great power, influence, wealth, or, of being a famous person. These seem to represent a regression to an earlier phase of development in which the child regards himself as omnipotent. An example is Don Quixote (Cervantes), whose Windmill Tilting was really his combat against the villainous foe.

4. Persecutory: Delusions in which the person feels watched, followed, slandered, vilified, or having his mind controlled or influenced by others, or, of being plotted against. An example is Captain Queeg, in *The Caine Mutiny* by Arthur Miller.

5. Litigious: Marked by disputatiousness, contentiousness or fondness for litigation or proneness to engage in lawsuits.

E. They show no other signs of mental illness aside from the delusional system. There is no withdrawal or regression as seen in schizophrenia, nor any affective changes as seen in manic-depressive illness.

F. In projection, inner unconscious feeling's become more acceptable in their externalized conscious form.

III. **Incidence**

A. Paranoid states account for about 10 percent of hospital admissions.

B. Recent studies indicate that they are about twice as common among women as among men.

C. The proportion of unmarried people in this group is higher than for the general population.

D. They are more common among immigrant groups and migratory people.

E. Classical paranoia (paranoia vera or true paranoia) is very rare.

IV. **Psychopathological factors**

A. The overuse of denial and projection as defenses against underlying conflicts, feelings of insecurity, reputiated impulses, or other conflictual factors.

B. As a child, the paranoiac was very likely suspicious, seclusive, secretive, and unable to develop any underlying basic trust.

C. As an adult, he is sensitive, distrustful, biased, and shows undue egocentricity (narcissism) and unyielding rigidity.

D. In those with graniose ideation, the behavior may be a response to needs for improving self-esteem or enhancing prestige.

E. In general, his prepsychotic personality would be characterized as a paranoid personality (hypersensitivity, rigidity, suspicion, jealousy, envy, excessive self-importance, and tendency to blame others and to ascribe evil motives to them).

F. Psychodynamically, there is projection of certain unacceptable impulses.
  1. According to Freud, these were repressed, homosexual drives.
  2. According to Adler, these were repressed inferiority feelings.
  3. These may be any type of repressed conflict, especially hostile and aggressive feelings.

G. Often the paranoid is of superior intellect.

H. A high percentage either don't marry or are divorced (perhaps because of hostile and homosexual strivings).

V. **Clinical syndromes:** The following conditions are listed as varieties of the paranoid states in the new nomenclature.
  A. Paranoia
  B. Involutional paranoid state (involutional paraphrenia)
  C. Other paranoid state

VI. **Other conditions with paranoid delusions:** There are other psychotic disorders which show paranoid delusions, such as paranoid schizophrenia, alcoholic paranoid state (alcohol paranoia), and certain psychoses associated with various organic brain syndromes. These are more properly classified elsewhere.

PARANOIA

Synonyms: true paranoia; paranoia vera

I. **Definition:** A psychotic disorder characterized by an elaborate, well-systematized, complex, intricate, logical, and well-fixed delusional system but with relatively good preservation of the remainder of the personality.

II. **Historical note**
  A. Literally the term, paranoia, means thinking beside one's self.

B. In antiquity the term *paranoia* was synonymous with the term *insanity.*

C. In the eighteenth century, it was used to describe delusional and delirious conditions.

D. Its present definition derives from the Kraepelinian classification.

III. Incidence

A. This is a rare psychosis although there may be some unrecognized cases because the delusional system is well disguised.

B. It is infrequent in youth because it is an insidiously developing condition which does not make itself obvious until later on.

C. It is most commonly diagnosed between the ages of twenty-five and forty.

IV. Psychopathology

A. In the classical psychoanalytic formulation, paranoia represents a regression to an early anal phase.

B. For further details see subsection on Etiology in the previous section.

V. Symptomatology

A. The principal symptoms are well-organized delusions (most commonly of persecution but sometimes of grandiosity).

B. Other symptoms are related to the patient's delusional system.

C. Characteristics of the delusion:
   1. Often concerns infidelity of the spouse or a plot against the patient's life.
   2. The patient commonly recognizes that others regard his idea as delusional, but he is not influenced by their opinion or by clear refutations.
   3. The delusion is not necessarily bizarre or even impossible. If one could accept the original premise, the remainder of the constructs appear reasonable and logical.
   4. Some paranoiacs keep their delusions hidden because they recognize that others regard them as psychotic symptoms.

D. The degree to which the individual may act on his delusion varies. He may only complain; he may become litigious; or he may become assaultive or homicidal. At best, he is a social nuisance; at worst, he may be a criminal.

VI. Prognosis

A. This is a chronic illness.

B. Prognosis for recovery is poor, though progression may halt at any stage of development.

C. Since there is relatively good preservation of the personality aside from the elaborate well-systematized delusional system, the patient's behavior is generally tolerated by society. Thus, most patients are never hospitalized but are regarded by others as "cranks" or eccentrics.

D. Sometimes with age there is a diminution in ability to follow through on the delusional system and hence, such people may become less of a nuisance.

VII. **Treatment**
   A. The delusions are unmodified by any known therapeutic technique.
   B. Most of the milder cases can make a marginal adjustment outside of the hospital, but a few cases eventually require institutionalization. Thus, it is best to try to attempt treatment while the patient remains in the community.
   C. The therapist who can accept the paranoiac, at the same time clearly indicating to him that he does not accept his delusional ideas, may be of value in a supportive way to the patient. Sometimes the person who is not skilled in dealing with such an individual may become a part of the patient's delusional system.
   D. Various psychotropic drugs, especially the phenothiazines, may be of some help in modifying the patient's delusional preoccupation or in assisting him to adapt more comfortably.
   E. Sometimes the management of such cases is determined more by the needs of society than by the needs of the individual patient.

INVOLUTIONAL PARANOID STATE

Synonym: involutional psychotic reaction; involutional paraphrenia

I. **Definition:** A paranoid psychosis with initial onset of delusion formation in the involutional period (late middle life).

II. **For discussion** of this disorder, the reader is referred to the section on involutional melancholia.

OTHER PARANOID STATE

Synonyms: paranoid condition; paranoid reaction; paraphrenia

I. **Definition:** An ill-defined group of reactions characterized by paranoid delusions which lack the logical systematization seen in paranoia but which do not show the regression and deterioration found in paranoid schizophrenia (this is a residual category for paranoid psychoses which are not classifiable elsewhere).

II. Paraphrenia
A. In the early nineteenth century, this term was used to describe a clinical syndrome, then known as *Folly* (schizophrenia).
B. Currently, the term is used to denote a disorder characterized by paranoid delusions without deterioration, dementia or loss of contact with reality, other than in the area of the delusional system.

III. Psychopathology (See section under "Paranoid States")

IV. Symptomatology
A. Delusions are not as well systematized as in paranoia and are often modifiable and shifting.
B. The patient does not act on the delusions in the persistent, militant fashion of the paranoiac.
C. Unlike paranoid schizophrenia, there is no evidence of personality deterioration.

V. Prognosis
A. The prognosis in these reactions is much more favorable than in paranoia, although these, too, may become recurrent or chronic.
B. Occasionally, some great stress will occasion an acute paranoid episode in an individual which subsides when the stress is removed.

VI. Treatment
A. Psychotherapy is often helpful in these conditions. The delusional symptoms are often responsive to therapeutic intervention.
B. Many times EST is helpful in shortening the duration of paranoid episodes.
C. Sometimes the major tranquilizers (especially the phenothiazines) may favorably influence delusional mentation.

VII. Case example:
Mr. H., a forty-year-old business executive, was admitted to the hospital mildly intoxicated and complaining that FBI agents were watching him because they suspected him of subversive activity. He had first developed ideas of suspiciousness ten years before while employed as an investigator for a governmental agency. Since that time, on several occasions, he had ideas that he was under surveillance by various investigating agencies.

These ideas were never well systematized, but he did react to them with great feeling; for example, he once planned to shoot himself to escape from the investigators. Often he would drink to allay the anxiety aroused by his paranoid ideas. These periods of paranoid ideation always responded well to treatment. Between such periods, he is somewhat sensitive and inclined to project but shows no withdrawal or personality deterioration. When he is well, he recognizes his tendency to project and the irrationality of his paranoid ideas.

In this case, note that his periods of illness were characterized chiefly by paranoid delusions but without hallucinations or inappropriate affect. The episodes responded well to treatment and between episodes he did not show any personality deterioration.

FOLIE À DEUX

I. **Definition:** A psychotic disorder in which two closely related people, usually members of the same family and who live in close intimate association, mutually share identical delusions.

II. **Introduction**
   A. This is a rare condition first described in 1877 by Laséque and Falret.
   B. It has sometimes been called double insanity or psychosis of association.
   C. Since it is usually paranoid in nature, it can be conveniently discussed with the paranoid states.
   D. Gralnick, who reviewed the English literature and reported on 103 cases in 1942, defined it as a "psychiatric entity characterized by the transference of delusional ideas or abnormal behavior from one person to one or more others who have been in close association with the primarily affected patient."

III. **Psychopathology**
   A. The essential psychological process is unconscious identification (A. Brill, 1920).
      1. There is a communication of delusional ideas from one person to another (both of whom have been closely associated for a long period of time).
      2. Frequently involves the parent and child, husband and wife, or two sisters.
      3. The identification is a mutual phenomenon.
      4. Nothing is ever accepted by the secondary partner that is ego-alien. That is, the delusional material from the primary

partner must resemble the unconscious fantasies and fit the defense mechanisms of the secondary partner.

    5. The identification in folie à deux may be more akin to identification with the aggressor. As this was described by Anna Freud, identification with the aggressor is a defensive maneuver which protects the ego against real or feared aggression by allowing the individual to share in the power of the feared one.

B. The interdependence of the two partners on each other is extreme and the identification is carried out in order to avoid separation which would be unendurable (H. Hartmann and E. Stengel, 1931).

C. In the prepsychotic relationship of the folie à deux pair, the primary or dominant partner is strongly dependent on the secondary partner and has few outside sources of gratifications.

D. The dominant individual (primary partner) in the relationship is usually the one who has the primary psychotic disorder, and the recipient (the secondary partner) of the induced delusions is often submissive, seclusive, and suspicious (i.e., schizoid), and develops these symptoms secondarily.

E. There is a close physical association between the two who have usually lived an existence in relative isolation and often in poverty. The dominant individual is usually intellectually brighter.

F. Since this disorder is usually characterized by delusions, the mechanism of projection is also operating. Because the primary partner is afraid of giving up the relationship, his emerging hostility must be defended against. The defense used is projection of the hostility onto an outsider as paranoid delusions—the result being a paranoid psychosis.

G. Usually both persons have a long history of poor adjustment.

IV. Treatment

A. Separation of the two involved individuals.

B. Psychiatric treatment directed at the dominant person (primary partner) who has the primary psychotic symptoms. Treatment modalities should follow those recommended for the particular paranoid condition which he has, including psychotherapy, hospitalization, tranquilizers, EST.

C. The recipient (secondary partner) may clear up without any formal treatment following separation from the primary psychotic partner.

V. Case example: A. T., a sixty-one-year-old single man, and V. T., his fifty-seven-year-old single sister with whom he had lived for many years, were referred to the court psychiatric consultant for evaluation after they had both been found guilty of violation of the city fire ordinance on a number of occasions. Their offense consisted in hoarding a number of combustible items and trash in their home and on their premises. Neighbors complained of this and the fire-prevention bureau, after repeatedly warning them about the combustible nature of the rubbish and other materials, filed a complaint. The man, on examination, showed flattened affect and was silly and inappropriate. He showed signs of schizoid behavior, including introversion, lack of spontaneity in his speech, blocking, and was overly sensitive and overly suspicious. The schizoid and paranoid elements in his personality were also evident in the pre-sentence study where it was learned that he tended to place much of the blame for the collection of rubbish on his sister with whom he lived. His Minnesota Multiphasic Personality Inventory profile was clearly psychotic, showing elevations of the scales on the right-hand side.

The sister, at the time of the examination, seemed quite frightened and kept asking during the examination whether her brother could not be present during the interview so he could "support me." She showed much preoccupation with her fantasy, but denied that she had hallucinations or delusions. She was evasive and defensive and had a number of "reasons" for the hoarding of the trash in their home. From her descriptions of the hoarding of the trash, she and her brother would apparently collect a number of items and then spend much time going over them to try sorting out things that might have some value. Whenever attempts were made to question her in detail about what valuable items might be in the trash or why the trash continued to accumulate, she would say, "You are trying to upset me."

Based on our examination, it was our impression that the brother was the one primarily ill and that he had a paranoid, schizophrenic reaction and that his sister also had the same psychotic illness, but because she was the passive, submissive, suggestible one, she had developed it secondarily, through induction.

REFERENCES

Freedman, A. M.; Kaplan, H. I.; and Saddock, Benjamin J. *Modern Synopsis of Comprehensive Textbook of Psychiatry*. Baltimore: Williams & Wilkins, 1972, chap. XIV.

Kolb, Lawrence C. *Modern Clinical Psychiatry.* 8th ed. Philadelphia: W. B. Saunders Company, 1973, chap. XXIII.

Pulver, S. E., and Brunt, M. Y. "Deflection of Hostility and Folie À Deux." *Archives of General Psychiatry* 5(1961):257-265.

It is—last stage of all—
When we are frozen up within, and quite
The phantom of ourselves,
To hear the world applaud the hollow ghost
Which claimed the living man.

Matthew Arnold, "Growing Old,"
New Poems, 1867

Organic Brain Syndromes

Synonyms: organic psychosis; toxic psychosis; toxic delirium; nonpsychotic organic brain syndromes

I. **Definition:** Mental disorder caused by or associated with impairment of brain tissue function.

II. **Characteristics of organic brain syndromes**
   A. The fundamental process is the destruction or damage of neurons (nerve calls).
   B. It is this damage rather than the quality of the destructive process that is responsible for the typical clinical picture.
   C. Strictly speaking, damage to the brain does not in itself fully account for the occurrence of the abnormal behavior. Psychological and sociocultural factors also play a role.
      1. Psychological factors: Previous personality; the manner in which he coped with environmental stresses and internal conflicts; the characteristic manner by which he deals with his organic deficit is determined by his adjustive patterns and coping mechanisms.
      2. Sociocultural factors: Includes the demands of the environment, the psychosocial setting in which the illness develops, the characteristics of his cultural background, the presence or absence of support from family and others.

D. Thus for example, senile changes in the brain may produce confusional and deteriotated behavior in one person, depressive symptoms in a second person, paranoid behavior in a third person, or have no appreciable affect on yet a fourth person.

E. The reactions in organic brain syndromes might be regarded as being released by the brain damage and superimposed upon it.

III. Occurrence

A. These reactions may occur at any age.

B. Some, such as senile reaction and cerebral arteriosclerosis, are found in late life. Others such as Pick's disease (a presenile degenerative disease of the brain affecting the cerebral cortex, particularly the frontal lobes) or Alzheimer's disease (a degenerative organic brain disease) are found in middle life. Others, such as head injuries, are more commonly found in early life. Also, toxic reactions associated with infectious diseases or alcoholic psychotic reactions, may occur at almost any age.

C. Some organic brain syndromes seem to be increasing in frequency, as for example, senile dementia and psychoses with cerebral arteriosclerosis (because of the aging population). Others are decreasing in frequency, as for example, psychosis with syphilis of the central nervous system (general paresis).

IV. Etiology

A. Any condition which produces cerebral tissue impairment may lead to the production of this syndrome. Included among the possible causes are the following: infections (interacranial and systemic), toxins, drugs, alcohol, brain trauma, circulatory disturbances, metabolic or nutritional disorder (such as uremia, diabetes, vitamin deficiencies, anemia), senile or presenile brain disease, intracranial neoplasms (either primary or metastatic), convulsive disorders, birth trauma, cerebral arteriosclerosis, and certain diseases of unknown or uncertain cause (such as multiple sclerosis, Huntington's chorea, Pick's disease, Alzheimer's disease), or any other degenerative disease of the central nervous system.

B. Actually, any disease or agent which produces central nervous system pathology may produce an organic brain syndrome.

C. The most common chronic organic brain syndromes seen in clinical practice are:

1. Senile dementia, or nonpsychotic organic brain syndrome with senile brain disease.

      2. Psychosis with cerebral arteriosclerosis, or nonpsychotic organic brain syndrome with cerebral arteriosclerosis.

  D. It has been estimated by Freedman et al. that about 10 to 15 percent of patients hospitalized on acute medical and surgical services manifest some degree of acute brain syndrome (delirium). Perhaps the most commonly seen ones would be those associated with drugs (e.g., general anesthesia, barbiturates, sedatives, etc.).

  E. Many acute brain syndromes, such as toxic deliria, never appear in statistical tables because they clear up rapidly under treatment on medical and surgical wards and are never transferred to psychiatric services for evaluation and treatment (e.g., an acute delirious reaction following cataract surgery in an elderly individual).

V. Symptomatology

  A. Most of these reactions, regardless of the specific etiology, are characterized by a basic syndrome consisting of the following:

      1. Impaired orientation (for time, place, or person).

      2. Impaired memory (memory for recent events is impaired before memory for remote events).

      3. Impaired judgment.

      4. Impaired intellectual functioning (knowledge, learning, comprehension, calculation, etc.)

      5. Lability and shallowness of affect.

  B. There is usually some evidence of the organic or toxic factor from the history, physical, neurological, or laboratory examinations. For example, peripheral arteriosclerosis in a person with cerebral arteriosclerosis; skull fracture in someone who has brain trauma; paralysis, paresis, reflex or sensory changes in cases with brain tumors; urinary or blood chemistry changes in people who have had heavy metal poisoning; evidence of cerebral atrophy on pneumoencephalographic X-ray studies in a person with Pick's or Alzheimer's disease; history of excessive alcoholic intake in someone with an alcoholic psychosis; history of exposure to some industrial toxin in acute brain syndrome.

  C. The brain syndromes are grouped into psychotic and nonpsychotic disorders according to the severity of the functional impairment.

      1. Psychoses associated with organic brain syndromes:

         a. A patient is psychotic when his mental functioning is sufficiently impaired to interfere grossly with his capacity to meet the ordinary demands of life.

      b. There may be serious reality distortion, including delusions and hallucinations and other types of perceptual distortions.

      c. There may be marked alterations in the mood leading to inappropriateness.

      d. There may be marked aggravation in the impairment syndrome.

  2. Nonpsychotic organic brain syndromes:

      a. Patients with this condition have evidence of organic brain syndrome but are not psychotic.

      b. The organic brain damage present does not significantly impair the patient's ability to meet the ordinary demands of living and his relationship with reality remains essentially intact.

D. Many times patients who are aware of their organic deficit will demonstrate denial, rationalization, and projection as defenses against facing the threatening implications of the cognitive loss.

E. In children, mild brain damage often manifests itself by hyperactivity, short attention span, easy distractability, and impulsiveness. Sometimes the child is withdrawn, restless, unresponsive, and may perseverate (DSM-II, page 31-32).

VI. Clinical types

A. Even though the current classification does not make a diagnostic distinction between *acute* and *chronic* brain syndromes, from the clinical point of view, it is important to distinguish these two types of brain disorders because of the marked differences in the course, prognosis, and treatment of the illnesses. The terms primarily indicate whether the brain damage and its accompanying organic brain syndrome is reversible (acute) or whether it is permanent and persistent (chronic). Some brain syndromes may occur in either form. Some occur only in acute forms and others only in chronic form. (DSM-II, page 22-23)

B. Acute brain syndromes

  1. These reactions are characterized by disorientation with confusion and often with hallucinations. They are produced by cerebral metabolic insufficiency and are often called deliria.

  2. Symptoms: In addition to the "impairment" symptoms listed under V, the patient typically shows:

      a. Obvious mood changes. Most commonly, he is anxious,

fearful or excited, although, he may show irritability, defensiveness or even rages.
   b. Motor behavior: Shows restlessness, clumsiness, difficulty in articulations, slurring of speech, perseveration, and decreased tolerance to alcohol.
   c. Hallucinations: These are vivid and frequently colorful. The details are clearly perceived by the patient and he reacts to them realistically. This partly explains some of the mood changes mentioned above (contrast these hallucinations with those present in schizophrenia).
   d. Delusions are common.
3. Etiology
   a. Any agent or affection which produces cerebral metabolic insufficiency which is temporary and reversible may cause acute brain syndrome. Thus, alcohol, infection, drugs, various toxins such as found in certain industries, head trauma, or certain metabolic disturbances (such as porphyria, uremia, diabetic acidosis, or coma), cardiac failure or arrest, respiratory failure, febrile illnesses, anemia as well as any disease in which the bodily homeostasis is seriously disrupted.
   b. The symptoms are not specifically related to the nature of the causal agent. All of the etiological factors mentioned under *a* can produce the same symptom picture.
   c. Since most these reactions are toxic in origin, this is a convenient place to list the types of toxins. Toxins are either exogenous or endogenous.
      (1) Exogenous toxins are developed outside of the body and are introduced into the body chiefly through ingestion or absorption. Examples are alcohol, bromides, barbiturates, some of the newer nonbarbiturate sedatives, opiates, hallucinogenic drugs, heavy metals (viz, lead, arsenic), or various industrial and commercial toxins.
      (2) Endogenous toxins are produced within the body in association with some physical illness. Examples are the toxins produced in delirious reactions associated with infectious disease of various types, uremia, diabetes, pernicious anemia.
4. Treatment
   a. This depends upon the underlying etiology.
   b. The general principles of treatment are:
      (1) Elimination of the toxin.

(2) Treatment of the underlying disease which precipitated the mental changes.
c. Supportive measures including nursing care, maintenance of nutrition, fluid intake, etc.
d. Either phenothiazines (thorazine, mellaric) or minor tranquilizers (valium, librium) and sedatives (for example, Chloral Hydrate, Dalmane, are often helpful).
e. Where organic brain damage is minor, reparative efforts may be extremely successful. This should be kept in mind in any rehabilitation program.

5. Prognosis is ordinarily good. Since the cerebral impairment is usually temporary and reversible, the patient usually recovers.

C. Chronic brain syndromes
1. Since these reactions result from more or less irreversible brain destruction, there is some permanent persistence of impairment symptoms and behavioral changes.
2. There is usually a history of long-term progression and worsening of the impairment symptoms (orientation, memory, judgment, intellectual functioning). In chronic brain syndrome there is a serious impairment in all spheres of cognition. (Mental processes of memory, reasoning, and judgement).
3. Etiology
a. Any illness or disorder which produces irreversible brain damage may cause chronic brain syndrome. Examples are cerebral arteriosclerosis; senility; Alzheimer's disease; Pick's disease; Huntington's chorea (a rare, progressive, degenerative disease occurring in families and characterized by choreic movements and progressive mental deterioration); alcohol; central nervous system syphilis; heavy metals; intracranial neoplasms; metabolic or endocrine disturbances, etc.
b. As noted under acute brain syndrome, the symptoms are not specifically related to the underlying etiology. All the disorders listed under *a* can produce the same "impairment" symptoms and personality changes.
4. Treatment is not very successful since the underlying disease is relatively permanent, more or less irreversible, and has produced a diffuse impairment of cerebral tissue function. General supportive measures, including nursing care, maintenance of fluid intake, nutrition, etc., are sometimes

helpful. Medications which produce cerebral vasodilitation are sometimes useful (nicotinic acid; Hydergine). Attempts should be made to care for such a person in his usual familiar surroundings for as long as possible. Avoidance of social isolation is important.

5. Prognosis is usually poor since the brain destruction is permanent. However, it should be remembered that the clinical course is not always progressive. Some individuals may show slight improvement and others may have a course characterized by exacerbations and remissions. It should be remembered that there are instances of massive brain damages which have not shown any clinically discernable signs of impairment.

VII. Case examples

A. Acute brain syndrome

1. A thirty-five-year-old man was admitted to the hospital for treatment of a leg injury. He gave a history of alcoholism dating back to age eighteen and said that he had been drinking at least one pint of whiskey daily for several months prior to admission. The morning following admission the nurses noted that he seemed confused and could not give the correct date or the name of the hospital. By late afternoon he appeared anxious and swept his hand along his trunk and extremities as if brushing something from him. On inquiry he admitted to "seeing" tiny green animals crawling over his body. By late evening he was very excited and fearful, especially if left by himself in the darkened room. He was transferred to the psychiatric ward where he recovered from the acute psychotic episode after two days.

   In this case, note the history of exposure to a toxin (chronic alcoholism), the sudden onset of "impairment" symptoms (disorientation, etc.), mood change, and the vivid, visual hallucinations. Note also the rapid recovery from the acute episode.

2. A seventy-four-year-old man developed symptoms of enlarged prostate (benign prostatic hyperthrophy), viz., frequent urination, nocturia, dysuria, and urinary retention. The urinary retention became so severe that he had to be hospitalized. Two days after admission he became confused, disoriented, and unruly. He admitted to visual hallucinations (e.g., he saw his son outside the sixth floor

hospital room) and was delusional (he was paranoid about some of the nurses and at times thought he was God). Examination revealed a markedly enlarged prostate gland and an elevated blood urea nitrogen (indicative of uremia). Following surgical resection of the enlarged prostate, his uremia cleared and his mental symptoms disappeared.

In this case, note that the symptoms are produced by an endogenous toxin (uremia) and disappear when this is cleared up by treating the underlying cause of the uremia.

B. Chronic brain syndrome
  1. A forty-eight-year-old woman was brought to the hospital by her son who said she was disoriented, showed poor judgment, was difficult to manage, and behaved in a childish manner. The onset of symptoms was noted two years earlier when she first complained of impaired memory for recent events and forgot some of the routine tasks associated with her job as a receptionist. Very shortly after this she showed poor judgment in dealing with people and frequently made obscene remarks to her fellow workers. Because of this behavior she was discharged from her job. At home her behavior showed progressive deterioration; she became slovenly in dress, was careless of excreta, and was markedly disoriented. At the time of admission she was incapable of carrying out even simple household tasks. Examination revealed her to be completely disoriented for time and place. Recent and remote memory were totally defective. Her behavior was characterized by apathy, disinterest, and passive cooperation. At times she seemed to be responding to auditory hallucinations. Physical and neurological examinations were essentially negative. A pneumoencephalogram (X-ray examination of the skull after replacing the cerebrospinal fluid with air) revealed findings compatible with generalized cerebral atrophy. She was transferred to a state hospital where her behavior has become progressively more deteriorated.

In this case, note the rather typical organic symptoms and the progressive nature of the symptoms resulting from the permanent and progressive cerebral atrophy. This generalized cerebral atrophy occurring in middle life is called Alzheimer's disease. The pathological changes in the brain are similar to those found in senile psychotic reactions.

2. A seventy-six-year-old widow was admitted to the hospital complaining of memory loss and hallucinations. She had been well until about one year earlier when her family first noticed that she was forgetful and had trouble remembering the date. Shortly after this she complained of hearing strange noises in her apartment. The family was not especially concerned by this complaint since they knew one of her neighbors had frequent parties, and another kept a dog and other pets in his apartment. About four months before admission the patient began complaining that her next-door neighbor was a gangster and accused him of shooting someone in his apartment. One week before admission she went to the manager of the apartment building and complained about the people who were walking through her closed doors and windows. Her family was summoned and they brought her to the hospital. Examination revealed her to be grossly disoriented for time and place. Both recent and remote memory were impaired. She admitted to visual hallucinations (e.g., she saw dogs in her room) and was mildly suspicious of the staff. Physical and neurological studies were negative except for X-ray evidence of mild rheumatoid arthritis. After a few weeks her hallucinations and delusions cleared up and she recognized that she had experienced a psychotic episode. At the time of discharge to her family two months later, she was still disoriented for time and had a fair amount of recent memory impairment. However, she was able to return to her apartment and adjust with only minimal supervision.

This is a senile psychotic reaction. Note the onset in late life of "impairment" symptoms followed by behavioral changes in the absence of any specific positive physical, neurological, or laboratory findings. The "improvement" following hospitalization is not unusual in this type of reaction, although as noted in this case, there is some residual of the permanent brain damage (disorientation and memory loss persisted after discharge).

REFERENCES

American Psychiatric Association. *Diagnostic and Statistical Manual of Mental Disorders*, 2nd ed. Washington, D.C., 1968. Seventh Printing, July 1974.

Freedman, A. M., Kaplan, H. I., and Saddock, B. J. *Modern Synopsis of Comprehensive Textbook of Psychiatry*. Baltimore: Williams & Wilkins Company, 1972, chap. XVII.

Kolb, L C. *Modern Clinical Psychiatry*. 8th ed. Philadelphia: W. B. Saunders Company, 1973, chap. IX-XIX.

Solomon, P., and Patch, V. D. *Handbook of Psychiatry*. 2nd ed. Los Altos, California: Lang Medical Publications, 1971, chap. XV.

False facts are highly injurious to
the progress of science, for they
often endure long; but false views,
if supported by some evidence,
do little harm, for every one takes
salutory pleasure in proving their falseness.

Charles Robert Darwin: DESCENT OF MAN,
1809-1892

Assessment of the Psychiatric Patient

By: Shirley H. Mink, Ph.D., and Walter D. Mink, Ph.D.

I. **Purposes of assessment:** Assessment procedures play an important role in establishing a working diagnosis and planning a treatment program for a psychiatric patient. Systematic assessment contributes to establishing the probable etiology and course of the patient's disorder, predicting his response to treatment, and evaluating results of treatment.

II. **Areas of investigation:** Assessment procedures elicit information about the following areas of the patient's condition and experience:
   A. Current psychological functioning and symptom formation.
   B. Current life situation and sources of stress.
   C. Personal history including critical developmental incidents.
   D. Personality structure and defenses (psychodynamics).

III. **Methods of assessment**
   A. The interview
      1. The interview is the most widely used assessment technique in psychiatric practice.
      2. The interview provides not only factual information about the patient, but also an opportunity to observe such personal characteristics as appearance, manner, speech, and mode of interpersonal response.

3. Interviews with informants other than the patient provide independent information which may corroborate the patient's report or may indicate important omissions and inconsistencies. This source of information is particularly important when patients may be without insight, delusional, confused, or otherwise inaccessible or uncooperative.

4. In psychiatric interviewing, the following points of inquiry are usually included:
   a. Presenting complaint
   b. History of present illness
   c. Nature of previous adjustment
   d. Educational, social, and occupational history
   e. Family and marital history
   f. Past medical history

B. Mental status examination: The mental status examination is a special form of assessment often conducted in conjunction with the history-taking interview. (Refer to section on symptom formation in mental disorders.) It provides an outline for recording objective descriptions of patient behavior as follows:

1. Mental content: The thoughts, concerns, and trends which are uppermost in the patient's mind; content disturbances include delusions, hallucinations, obsessions, and phobias.

2. Sensorium and intellect: The degree of the patient's awareness and level of functioning; disturbances of orientation, memory, retention, attention, information, and judgment can be elicited with standardized questions and test materials.

3. Stream of thought (speech): Quantitative and qualitative aspects of the patient's communication; disturbances include over- and underproductivity, disconnectedness, unintelligibility, and incoherence.

4. Emotional tone (mood or affect): Patient's report of subjective feelings and examiner's objective observations of facial expression, posture, and attitude; disturbances include quantitative deviations (elation, depression, apathy) and incongruence among subjective report, behavioral observation, and mental content.

5. Attitude, manner and behavior: Appearance, dress, facial expression, activity, posture, and general interview and ward demeanor; disturbances include deviations of degree of activity, mannerisms, distortions of motility, and uncooperativeness.

6. Insight: The degree to which the patient can appreciate the nature of his condition and need for treatment.
7. Instruments have been developed to standardize the mental status examination. The Mental Status Schedule is an example of such an instrument. In this test a trained interviewer administers a mental status examination guided by a standard interview schedule and scores the responses objectively at intervals during the session. The Inpatient Multidimensional Psychiatric Scale provides a systematic way for rating the behavior of severely disturbed psychiatric patients.

C. Physical and neurological examination: A routine physical and neurological examination is an essential part of general psychiatric assessment. Special diagnostic and laboratory procedures are used when there is suspicion of organic involvement.

D. Psychological testing: The next section provides a detailed outline of psychological testing procedures in psychiatric assessment.

IV. **Psychological testing:** The development of psychological measurement of human characteristics has provided many tools that are of particular value in psychiatric assessment.

A. Variability from person to person is a commonly acknowledged aspect of many characteristics of human behavior. Psychological testing is based on the assumption that differences in these characteristics can be measured.

B. Technically, a test is a systematic procedure of obtaining samples of behavior for the comparison of two or more persons.

C. The development, administration, and interpretation of the tests most widely used in psychiatric assessment require special skill and training. The American Psychological Association has established ethical standards for the distribution and use of psychological tests.

D. Criteria for evaluation of psychological tests: While psychological tests vary in content, purpose and range of application, the evaluation of tests should consider the following characteristics:

1. Reliability: Refers to the consistency with which a test measures what it proposes to measure.
2. Validity: Refers to the accuracy with which a test fulfills its purpose of prediction, selection, or classification.
3. Standardization: Refers to the establishment of norm

groups which permit the comparison of an individual test result to an appropriate reference group.

E. Other characteristics of tests:
1. Form of administration: Some tests can be administered to only one person at a time (individual tests); others can be given to any number of persons at one time (group tests).
2. Standardization of administration: Tests vary in the degree to which the tester must follow a prescribed procedure in the administration of the test.
3. Objectivity: Tests vary in the degree to which interpretation is required in the scoring of responses. An objective test is one which is scored in a standardized way which minimizes differences among different scorers.
4. Form of response: Some tests require a specific form of response (e.g., true-false); others permit open-end responses (e.g., sentence completion).

F. Commonly used tests in psychiatric assessment:
1. Intelligence tests
   a. The "intelligence" measured by intelligence tests is considered to be a general, relatively stable capacity to learn and deal effectively with one's environment.
   b. Intelligence is assumed to be normally distributed in the population.
   c. The results of intelligence tests are frequently reported in terms of an IQ (intelligence quotient) score.
   d. The IQ score indicates the position of a person's intelligence test performance relative to the average performance of his age group. The average IQ is 100.
   e. The commonly used classification of intelligence is as follows: Very Superior—IQ 130 and above; Superior—120-129; Bright-Normal—110-119; Average—90-109; Dull-Normal—80-89; Borderline—70-79; Mental Defective—69 and below.
   f. In psychiatric practice, the intelligence test has the following main uses:
      (1) To aid in establishing the diagnosis of mental retardation.
      (2) To assess the effects of brain damage.
      (3) To assess effective intellectual performance in psychiatric disorders.
      (4) To define a patient's intellectual resources for educational and vocational adjustment.

g. Since "intelligence" is, to a substantial degree defined culturally, tests of intelligence reflect competencies and achievements which are considered important for success in the culture; interpretations of tests results should be made with full consideration of the appropriateness of the test for the particular person who is tested.

h. Major intelligence tests in current usage

(1) The New Revised Stanford-Binet (1960) is a widely used, individually administered intelligence test for children and for the assessment of mental retardation, and has served as the standard for comparison with other tests of intellectual ability.

(a) The test is composed of various tasks and problems organized by year levels arranged from two years to superior adults.

(b) The problems successfully solved at each year level are totalled and the sum is expressed as a Mental Age Score and has an IQ score equivalent.

(c) Examples of types of tasks included are vocabulary, memory span for digits, words, and sentences, reasoning, comprehension, copying geometric figures, etc.

(d) Verbal ability is strongly emphasized in this test, and it has proved useful in the prediction of school achievement.

(e) The test is of limited usefulness with adults because it was standardized primarily with children and is composed of tasks which are more appropriate for children.

(f) It is the test of choice for reliable assessment of the extreme ranges of intelligence, both low and high.

(2) The Wechsler Adult Intelligence Scale (WAIS) is the most widely used individually administered intelligence test for adults and is the standard against which other adult intelligence tests are compared.

(a) The test is composed of a series of subtests organized into a Verbal Scale and a Performance Scale. The verbal subtests are Information, Comprehension, Similarities, Arithmetic, Digit Span, Vocabulary. Performance subtests are Picture Arrangement, Picture Completion,

Block Design, Object Assembly, and Digit Symbol.

(b) The test yields three IQ scores: Verbal Scale IQ, Performance Scale IQ, and Full Scale IQ.

(c) Differences between verbal and performance IQ scores may sometimes be of diagnostic value. However, differences in the pattern of subtest scores have not proved to be of any consistent diagnostic significance.

(d) Two other forms of the Wechsler Intelligence Scale exist: Wechsler-Bellevue Form I (which is now rarely used) and Wechsler-Bellevue Form II which is the retest instrument for the WAIS.

(e) Two forms of the test have also been developed for children. The Wechsler Intelligence Scale for Children (WISC) is designed for children ages five to fifteen, and is the most widely used intelligence test for children. The Wechsler Pre-School and Primary Scale of Intelligence (WPPSI) has been developed for children ages four to six and one-half.

(3) Special individually administered intelligence tests have been devised for use with illiterate, blind, deaf, and other handicapped persons who would not be accurately tested on the standard tests.

(4) Group tests: Large numbers of paper and pencil group tests of intelligence are available and are used primarily in schools and personnel departments in business and industry. While these tests generally yield an IQ score, it may be more meaningful to reserve the use of the term IQ for the individually administered intelligence test.

2. Personality tests
   a. There is a great variety of personality measures which differ in form, content, and interpretation.
   b. Some personality measures attempt to assess personality traits or characteristics; others attempt to reveal a pattern of personality dynamics (motives, defenses, conflicts, etc.).
   c. Personality measures can be classified roughly as objective tests and as projective techniques.
      (1) Objective tests
         (a) Objective tests usually take the form of ques-

tionnaires or rating scales in which the patient responds to the items according to how characteristic they are of his experience and behavior.

(b) Tests are administered and scored in a standardized way with the results expressed in numerical scores.

(c) Since objective tests are a form of self-report, they are open to faking and dissimulation. Ease of administration permits testing of large numbers of persons in a way which does not require special clinical personnel.

(d) The Minnesota Multiphasic Personality Inventory (MMPI)

1' This is the most widely used objective personality test in psychiatric practice.

2' The MMPI consists of 550 true-false items.

3' Validity scales: Four special scales are scored which indicate response tendencies and test-taking attitudes which might make interpretations of the test doubtful.

4' Clinical scales: Responses are scored in terms of correspondence to the responses of diagnosed psychiatric groups (hypochondriasis, depression, hysteria, psychopathic deviate, masculinity-femininity, paranoia, psychasthenia, schizophrenia, hypomania, and social introversion).

5' In addition to the clinical scales, many research scales have been developed for special purposes or to measure other personality characteristics (e.g. dependency, ego-strength, etc.).

6' Interpretation of the test is based on the pattern of scale scores. In recent years, standardized interpretations have been developed for common patterns. Computer systems have been devised which not only score the test, but can produce analyses of profiles.

7' A sizable research literature (more than 3,000 articles and books) has been developed around the MMPI. Reviews of this literature indicate that this test is reliable and valid for many uses.

(2) Projective techniques

    (a) Characteristics of projective measures.

        1' The materials of most projective methods are unstructured or ambiguous and require that the patient organize them in some imaginative way. The term *projective* implies that the patient "projects" his personality into the responses he gives.

        2' The patient has considerable freedom in his response.

        3' It is assumed that the way in which the patient responds reveals emotional and motivational factors which are characteristic of him, though perhaps on an unconscious basis.

        4' Interpretation of responses is subjective and is usually based on the theoretical assumptions of the interpreter. This leads to a lower degree of consistency from interpreter to interpreter than is obtained with objective tests.

        5' Both the administration and interpretation of projective techniques require special training and experience.

    (b) The Rorschach method

        1' The Rorschach is the best known and most widely used of the projective techniques.

        2' The materials consist of ten "ink blots." The patient is asked to describe what each card looks like. He may give as many responses to each card as he can.

        3' Following this administration of the test, the examiner conducts an inquiry, asking the subject to indicate the location of each response and to tell what about the blot (e.g., shape, color, and/or texture) contributed to the response.

        4' Responses are scored according to content (e.g., human, animal, object, X-ray, etc.), the area of the blot included in the content (whole blot or a particular section of it), and the characteristics of the blot (e.g., color, shading, and shape) which determine the content.

5' Interpretation is based on assumed personal significance of the responses, as well as characteristic ways in which the patient organizes his responses. A developing theory of Rorschach responses relates such factors as the use of color and the interpretation of movement to forms of psychopathology. Interpretation rests heavily on psychoanalytic theory, especially Jungian Theory.

6' A tremendous literature (more than 3,000 articles and books) pertaining to the Rorschach has developed. Reviews of this literature consistently raise serious questions about the reliability and validity of this instrument.

(c) The Thematic Apperception Test (TAT)

1' This procedure consists of twenty illustrations. The patient is asked to tell a story about the content of each picture.

2' Several complete methods of scoring have been developed which require special training in their use.

3' Stories are interpreted in terms of their themes, the handling of motivational states, and the resolution of conflicts, the ways in which interpersonal relations are presented, and the extent to which the patient identifies himself with the characters he describes.

(d) Other projective techniques: A large number of other techniques involving word association, sentence completion, drawing, and storytelling have been devised. They have in common the assumption that imaginative productions and fantasy yield important clues to personality organization.

3. Vocational interest and aptitude tests

a. Since the problems faced by some patients involve vocational maladjustment and dissatisfaction, vocational

testing can contribute important information to a total
treatment program.
  b. Aptitude tests
    (1) Tests are available which measure a variety of spe-
        cial aptitudes and abilities such as clerical ability,
        mechanical ability, spatial reasoning, hand and
        finger dexterity, and rate of manipulation.
    (2) Norms permit comparison of individual scores with
        scores of representative occupational groups.
    (3) The assessment of aptitudes for professional and
        managerial occupations is more complex and in-
        volves also the measurement of a combination of
        intellectual, personality, and interest factors.
  c. Interest tests
    (1) Interest tests are constructed to permit the compari-
        son of individual response patterns with the re-
        sponse patterns of persons representative of a
        number of professions and occupations.
    (2) The most commonly used vocational interest test for
        adults is the Strong Vocational Interest Blank
        (SVIB).
    (3) Interest test scores have been shown to be strongly
        related to job satisfaction.
4. Brain damage tests
  a. The assessment of intellectual deficit and the differenti-
      ation of organic brain conditions is often a problem in
      psychiatric diagnosis.
  b. The most accurate assessment of deficit due to brain
      damage can be made if earlier test performances are
      available with which comparisons can be made. In prac-
      tice, this is seldom possible.
  c. Some tests have been developed which compare per-
      formance on tasks sensitive to brain damage (e.g., ab-
      stract reasoning) with performance on tasks less af-
      fected by brain damage (e.g., vocabulary).
  d. Other tests have been designed which assess specific
      aspects of brain function such as memory, perception,
      language use, and motor coordination.
  e. At present, tests of brain damage sometimes yield help-
      ful diagnostic hypotheses. However, the eventual utility
      of tests of specific brain function is dependent on the
      success of current coordinated research into the neuro-
      logical and behavioral correlates of brain activity.

REFERENCES

American Psychological Association. *Standards for Educational and Psychological Tests and Manuals.* Washington, D.C.: American Psychological Association, 1966.

Buros, Oscar Kirsen, ed. *The Seventh Mental Measurements Yearbook.* Highland Park, New Jersey: The Gryphon Press, 1972.

Cranbach, L. *Essentials of Psychological Testing.* New York: Harper & Row, 1960.

Hathaway, S. R., and Meehl, P. E. *An Atlas for the Clinical Use of the MMPI.* Minneapolis: University of Minnesota Press, 1951.

Holtzman, W. H., Thorpe, J. S., Swartz, J. O., and Herron, E. W. *Inkblot Perception and Personality,* Austin: University of Texas Press, 1961.

Klopfer, B., and Kelly, D. M. *The Rorschach Technique.* New York: Harcourt, Brace & World, 1946.

Murray, H. A. et al. *Explorations in Personality.* New York: Oxford University Press, 1938.

Terman, L. L., and Merrill, M. A. *Measuring Intelligence.* Boston: Houghton Mifflin Company, 1937.

Wechsler, David. *The Measurement and Appraisal of Adult Intelligence, 14th Edition.* Baltimore: Williams & Wilkins Company, 1958.

———. *Wechsler Adult Intelligence Scale Manual.* New York: The Psychological Corporation, 1955.

———. *WISC Manual. Wechsler Intelligence Scale for Children.* New York: The Psychological Corporation, 1949.

Welsh, George Schlager, and Dahlstrom, W. Grant, eds. *An MMPI Handbook, A Guide to Use in Clinical Practice and Research.* Minneapolis: University of Minnesota Press, 1960.

———. *Basic Readings on the MMPI in Psychology and Medicine.* Minneapolis: University of Minnesota Press, 1956.

Canst thou not minister to a mind diseas'd;
Pluck from the memory a rooted sorrow;
Raze out the written troubles of the brain;
And, with some sweet oblivious antidote,
Cleanse the staff'd bosom of that perilous
    matter
Which weighs upon the heart?

Shakespeare: MACBETH

Treatment In Psychiatry

I. Introduction

A. Although something was mentioned about treatment of the various clinical syndromes in each section throughout the Outline, an attempt is made here to list in one place the various types of therapy that are used in psychiatry.

B. Much treatment in psychiatry has been empirical and has not been actually scientifically evaluated. In recent years there have been more attempts to accurately measure the effects of various therapies (e.g., there are reports of the effects of the various somatic and pharmacological therapies on emotional illnesses in which controls have been used; there have been attempts to scientifically evaluate the effects of psychotherapy).

C. Treatment in psychiatry can be grouped into five broad divisions:

1. Psychotherapy
2. Somatic therapy
3. Pharmacotherapy
4. Management therapy
5. Behavior therapy

II. Psychotherapy

A. In the broad sense this includes everything done to or for a patient that has a favorable effect upon him.

B. In the more traditional sense, psychotherapy is "the generic term for any type of treatment which is based primarily upon verbal or nonverbal communication with the patient as distinguished from the use of drugs, surgery, or physical measure such as electroconvulsive treatment."[1]

C. Types of psychotherapy: Psychotherapy can be conveniently divided into four types:
   1. Supportive psychotherapy
   2. Uncovering psychotherapy (intensive psychotherapy; genetic-dynamic therapy)
   3. Group psychotherapy
   4. Family therapy

D. Psychiatrists more or less agree on the aims of psychotherapy but are less generally agreed upon what psychotherapy is able to accomplish.

E. What type of patient will benefit from psychotherapy is not always clearly defined. Most people with neuroses and some with functional psychoses are considered candidates for psychotherapy. If there is no response to psychotherapy, some other form of treatment, such as pharmacotherapy or somatic therapy, may be recommended.

F. Of major importance in psychotherapy is the therapist-patient relationship.
   1. Rapport: "In psychiatry, the constant feeling of harmonious accord, mutual responsiveness and sympathy that contributes to the patient's confidence in the therapist and willingness to work cooperatively with him."[2]
      a. Rapport is important in any treatment relationship with the patient and regardless of whether or not the physician is treating him for an emotional or a physical illness.
      b. It is probably the singly most effective therapeutic tool that a physician has.
   2. Transference: The unconscious attachment to the therapist (or others who have a treatment relationship with the patient) of feelings and attitudes that were originally related to important figures (parents, siblings, etc.) in one's early life.

---

[1]American Psychiatric Association, *A Psychiatric Glossary* (New York: Springer Publishing Co.: 1968), p. 81.
[2]Ibid., p. 82.

3. Countertransference: The therapist's unconscious or conscious emotional reaction to the patient.
   a. It is important that the therapist recognize his countertransference feelings, especially the negative ones.
   b. Sometimes countertransference feelings can be used diagnostically and therapeutically. For example, irritability or hostility in the therapist may be induced by fear in the patient, and if the therapist is aware of his own countertransference feelings, he may more directly and correctly help the patient identify the underlying conflicts.
4. Both positive and negative feelings are involved in the transference and countertransference.

G. Psychotherapeutic technique is mainly influenced by the therapist's theoretical orientation. Reference is made to the various conceptions of personality development in psychodynamic formulations outlined in the chapter on Dynamic Concepts.

III. **Supportive psychotherapy:** Deals predominantly with conscious material and is centered chiefly on support of the individual's strength and assets. It is based primarily on the therapist-patient relationship. It includes:

A. Reassurance: The imparting or restoration of confidence and freeing the patient from fear and anxiety. It does not mean *false* reassurance. Examples:
1. Various physical and laboratory examinations which may relieve a person's anxiety about the significance of certain physical symptoms.
2. Psychological reassurance: For example, assuring one who fears serious mental illness that he will not lose his mind; or assuring a young mother that the hostile and aggressive thoughts she occasionally has toward her youngster are not signs of abnormality.

B. Ventilation (unburdening): The therapeutic release of feelings through conscious, free expression. This is "getting it off his chest." It serves two purposes: (1) sharing, this helps "dilute" the feelings and (2) self-punishment, from "revealing" one's self. For example: The sixty-year-old woman who was finally able to relate to the doctor how she had been emotionally clutching onto her thirty-five-year-old married daughter. After unburdening this fact, she was able to take the first major steps to release the hold on her daughter.

C. Environmental modification (environmental manipulation): This means changing the environment in any way. Caution must be exercised lest this type of treatment be misused. Examples:
  1. Providing a homemaker or housekeeper temporarily for a mother who has anxiety symptoms aggravated by the responsibilities of her children.
  2. Placing a patient in the relatively "neutral" environment of the hospital.
  3. Advising a vacation period away from home for a husband who has unduly prolonged grief reaction following the death of his wife.
  4. Persuading a spouse to modify behavior and attitudes if the patient for some reason is unable to do this.
D. Clarification: A process by which the physician helps the patient better understand his feelings and behavior and to have a clearer picture of external realities. Examples:
  1. Pointing out to an agitated and depressed patient that hospitalization will not make him worse.
  2. Pointing out to a paranoid patient that he projects. (This must be done in terms that are understandable to the patient.)
  3. Pointing out to a wife the rejecting behavior of her spouse who is really seeking a dissolution of the marriage.

IV. **Uncovering psychotherapy** (intensive psychotherapy, insight therapy): The aim is to produce insight through uncovering conflicts, chiefly unconscious, and learning to deal with them more effectively.
  A. The transference and countertransference phenomena are particularly important in this type of psychotherapy.
  B. This type of treatment includes psychoanalytic therapy and psychobiological therapy (distributive analysis).
    1. Psychoanalytic therapy: The exploration of the unconscious, chiefly through free association. Dream material is often evaluated for clues to unconscious feelings. Resistance (the opposition of the patient to facing his conflicts) must be recognized and dealt with.
    2. Psychobiological therapy: Critical examination and evaluation of conscious forces in the patient's personality development and emotional problems (i.e., he attempts to analyze, consciously, and synthesize).
    3. In many cases of emotional illness, both approaches may be

combined. As a matter of fact, most psychotherapists use an eclectic (the best from different systems) approach combining psychoanalytic as well as psychobiological techniques.

C. Hypnotherapy: Some psychiatrists use hypnosis as a means of facilitating psychotherapy. Occasionally hypnosis is employed to remove symptoms of psychogenic etiology (such as acute hysterical symptoms).

D. Examples of uncovering therapy:

1. A forty-five-year-old widower complained of impotence. After three psychotherapeutic interviews it was obvious that his symptom resulted from two important factors: his guilt about rejection of his wife because she was physically unattractive was reactivated when he was sexually aroused and his impotence was a protection against a second marriage to an aggressive woman he was dating but did not wish to marry. In this case, the conflicts were relatively superficial and readily accessible to the therapist. His symptom cleared when he recognized the dynamic factors and broke off his relationship with the woman.

2. A twenty-five-year-old man had consulted many physicians for palpitation, tachycardia, precordial pain, and apprehension. Each time physical and laboratory examinations revealed no evidence of cardiac disease. Although he worried about his heart, his symptoms were typical of anxiety reaction. In the first interview, it was apparent that his symptoms were related to his feelings about his father, but it was not until he had been seen for twelve sessions that he was able to see the relationship between his own anxiety symptoms and his father's heart attack one year earlier. When he did see that the onset of his own symptoms followed his father's heart attack and that his anxiety symptoms were really perpetuated by his guilt from some unconscious death wishes he had toward his father, his symptoms disappeared.

   The conflict in this case was not as superficial as in the previous case but was readily accessible to uncovering technique.

3. A thirty-year-old housewife had repeated episodes of parathesias, dizziness, and pains in her arms. These had begun shortly after her marriage and seriously handicapped her. After about fifty hours of psychotherapy, she was able to recognize that these symptoms always developed in

situations where she felt rejected by her husband. This rejection produced in her the same underlying feelings that she had as a result of her father's rejection of her during her early life. When she recognized this, her symptoms cleared.

The conflict here was unconscious and hence not as immediately available. Uncovering therapy brought the conflict to light.

V. **Group psychotherapy:** In this type of treatment, several individuals take part. It makes use of psychotherapeutic techniques in the group setting, including the utilization of group interaction. Usually there is one therapist and three or more patients. Although it is sometimes used alone, most commonly it is used in conjunction with individual psychotherapy and other types of psychiatric treatment.

A. This type of psychotherapy has its origins in observations made by Sigmund Freud in 1919 concerning the dynamics of the interplay between different individuals in a group setting. There is a definite pattern of interaction between the various members of a group which facilitates a therapeutic process. The group provides an opportunity for developing personal insights, as well as testing out new methods of coping and relating in a controlled type of environment.

B. There was a time when group psychotherapy was considered an expedient form, a way in which to involve a greater number of patients, but this is no longer felt to be true. For many patients it is superior to individual psychotherapy. The techniques closely parallel those of individual psychotherapy and depend upon the aims of the therapist and the type of patients. That is, groups may be conducted according to the psychoanalytic model of the nonparticipating therapist or the very active type of therapist as we see in counselling with all of the possible variants in between.

C. In the past decade a number of variations of group therapy have emerged which emphasize the use of group social processes in increasing self-understanding, improving relationships, and developing human potential; such procedures can be useful adjuncts to psychiatric treatment.

D. The variety of group procedures that are available to the public currently may be quite confusing to many people; no definitive "Consumer's Guide" is available so care should be exercised in evaluating the appropriateness of a group involvement for oneself.

VI. Family therapy

A. During the past several years, family therapy has been developed as a direct approach to the mental health of the family as an interacting unit.

B. In family therapy, emotional disturbances in individual members are seen as outgrowths of interpersonal conflicts between family members. The family unit is conceived of as a behavior system with unique properties of its own.

C. The focus is on the family with one or more therapists dealing with an entire family unit during the therapeutic sessions. The goal of treatment is to resolve or reduce the pathogenic conflicts and anxiety within the unit.

D. This is still an experimental treatment. In certain experimental situations, entire family units have been hospitalized in order to study the genesis of schizophrenia and other emotional disorders.

E. It may be used as the sole treatment or it may be used in conjunction with other types of therapy. It has been recommended for marital conflict and child-parent conflict situations.

F. Dr. Nathan Ackerman is a leading proponent of this type of therapy.

VII. Somatic therapy

A. History
 1. Modern somatic therapy in psychiatry began in about 1933 when Sakel first reported on the use of insulin coma therapy (hypoglycemic coma) in the treatment of mental disease.
 2. In 1936, von Meduna described metrazol convulsive therapy. This treatment was based on the erroneous assumption that schizophrenic symptoms and epilepsy were mutually antagonistic. This treatment has been largely abandoned.
 3. In 1938, Cerletti and Bini introduced electroconvulsive therapy. It replaced pharmacological convulsive therapy (metrazol convulsive therapy) and has remained an important treatment in psychiatry up to the present.

B. The chief somatic therapies are
 1. Electroshock therapy (electroconvulsive therapy)

a. There is no theory that satisfactorily explains the mode of action. It is important to remember that it is a symptomatic treatment (i.e., it does not treat underlying causes).

b. Technique: Sufficient electrical current is passed through electrodes applied to both temporal areas of the head to produce a grand mal seizure. A series of such treatments is given, the average being six to twelve. In recent years, certain medications have been given in conjunction with the treatment to minimize the apprehension and the physical risk. These drugs include:

(1) Atropine: To reduce salivation and inhibit vagal action.

(2) Succinylcholine chloride ("anectine"): To modify the muscular contractions of the convulsive seizures.

(3) Sedatives: Usually pentothal sodium or brevital (intravenously) to put the patient to sleep just prior to the treatment. Some physicians use oral barbiturates instead of intravenous pentothal prior to the treatment.

(4) The administration of the foregoing medications has reduced the apprehensions and physical risk to a bare minimum.

c. Indications

(1) Any depression will respond to EST but its use is sometimes limited to psychotic depressions or refractory depressive neuroses.

(2) Involutional melancholia seems to be a specific indication.

(3) EST shortens the periods of elation in manic-depressive illness.

(4) Acute schizophrenic episodes usually respond well to EST.

(5) It is important to remember that EST does not insure against relapse.

d. Contraindications: The physical risk is extremely low, particularly when given with the medications listed under "Technique." There are many physical conditions which were thought to increase the risk of the treatment, but with increased experience the number of physical conditions that contraindicate EST has dwindled to a bare minimum. Cases must be judged on an individual basis, however, weighing the possibility of psychiatric recovery against any possible physical risk.

2. Regressive electroshock therapy (R.E.S.T.; intensive electroshock therapy)
   a. This is a much more intensive course of treatment than the standard course of EST.
   b. Technique: Two or three grand mal convulsions are given daily until "regression" has occurred (marked confusion, memory loss, disorientation, lack of verbal spontaneity, a slurring of speech, and apathy; in other words, the patient behaves like a helpless infant—with bowel and bladder incontinence and a need to be fed). In some instances the treatments are terminated short of this point.
   c. Much nursing care is required if traditional R.E.S.T. is given. However, in intensive EST the patient may not require nearly so much nursing care.
   d. Indications: Certain cases of schizophrenia including pseudoneurotic schizophrenia (undifferentiated schizophrenia). Some also believe such treatment should be considered for anyone who is regarded as a candidate for psychosurgery.
3. Insulin coma therapy
   a. This is a serendipitous treatment for which there is no satisfactory explanation.
   b. Technique: Regular insulin is injected daily in increasing doses until hypoglycemic coma results. The period of coma is lengthened stepwise from ten to fifteen minutes up to one hour. Coma is terminated by administering glucose followed by food containing large amounts of protein. Usually a series of twenty-five or more comas is given.
   c. Indications: The chief indication for this type of treatment was severe, chronic schizophrenia.
   d. Contraindications: Diabetes mellitus, heart disease, pregnancy.
   e. This treatment has been used much less since the introduction of intensive EST.
4. Combined insulin-convulsive treatment
   a. In the past, ICT and EST have sometimes been used in combination in treating refractory cases which have shown poor response, or incomplete response, to either treatment alone.

    b. Various ways of combining the two have been recommended. For example:

      (1) Giving ICT and EST on alternating days.

      (2) A course of one treatment followed by a course of the other treatment.

      (3) Summation: This is giving a convulsion during the height of hypoglycemia.

    c. This treatment also is much less used since the introduction of intensive EST.

5. Narcoanalysis (or narcosynthesis): Occasionally a patient is interviewed under intravenously administered barbiturates. This may be helpful in removing certain symptoms which have been produced by acute traumatic situations.

6. Psychosurgery: This is a group of surgical procedures directed at certain areas of the brain in an effort to relieve various symptoms of mental illness. Included are the following:

    a. Frontal (prefrontal) lobotomy: This is the most commonly used of the psychosurgical procedures and consists of sectioning the frontal lobes of the brain. Two techniques are used:

      (1) Standard lobotomy: Here the surgical approach is made from above through holes in the skull.

      (2) Transorbital lobotomy: A specially designed instrument (leukotome) is inserted into the upper conjunctival sac and gently tapped through the orbital roof and the frontal lobes are sectioned from below.

    b. Bimedial, bilateral interior medial, and unilateral lobotomy have also been suggested as different surgical approaches.

    c. Frontal lobectomy: This is similar to lobotomy except that the frontal lobes are removed after sectioning. It does not have any advantage over lobotomy.

    d. Bilateral topectomy and undercutting: Selective partial ablation of the frontal cortex. Mostly, this procedure has been abandoned because it is technically difficult and has been followed by a high incidence of post-operative convulsions.

    e. Bilateral thalamotomy: A stereotaxic procedure in which portions of the dorsomedial nucleus of the thalamus are destroyed. A specially designed apparatus is necessary to perform this procedure.

f. Temporal lobotomy: Amputation of the anterior portion of the temporal lobes. Originally devised as a treatment for psychomotor epilepsy but has also been employed as a treatment in certain psychotic disorders.

g. Parietal and occipital lobotomies: These have been reported but the procedures have never become popular.

h. It should be kept in mind that these psychosurgical procedures are radical therapies and are used only as a "last resort" when other methods have failed.

VIII. Pharmacotherapy

A. Psychotherapeutic drugs have been available in the United States since 1954. Phenothiazine derivatives (one form of tranquilizers) were first introduced in France in 1952 and introduced into the United States in 1954. Rauwolfia derivatives had been used for centuries in India for many illnesses including mental illness.

B. The drugs in this group include
   1. Tranquilizers
   2. Antidepressants
   3. Lithium carbonate

C. Tranquilizing drugs

   1. These drugs produce tranquilization which is somewhat different from sedation.
   2. Tranquilization is the production of emotional calmness and relaxation without sedation, hypnosis, motor impairment, or euphoria. Tranquilizers act principally on the lower brain centers (in contrast to sedatives which act on the cortical areas as well).
   3. Classification of tranquilizers[3]
      a. Major tranquilizers: This group possesses the following characteristics:
         (1) They produce emotional calmness and mental relaxation.
         (2) They are highly effective in controlling symptoms of acutely and chronically disturbed psychotic patients.
         (3) They are capable of producing the reversible "extrapyramidal" syndrome (rigidity, tremors, drooling).

[3]W. M. Benson and B. C. Schiele, *Tranquilizing and Antidepressant Drugs,* (Springfield, Illinois: Charles C. Thomas, Publisher, 1962).

    (4) Produce a relatively high incidence of annoying side reactions.

    (5) Produce little, if any, habituation or dependency.

b. Minor tranquilizers: This group has the following characteristics:

    (1) Produce calmness and relaxation but of a different quality than the major tranquilizers.

    (2) Are not highly effective in the disturbed psychotic reactions but are helpful in relieving anxiety and tension.

    (3) They do not produce extrapyramidal phenomena.

    (4) Annoying side reactions are relatively rare.

    (5) Habituation may occur with some of these drugs.

c. List of major tranquilizers (most commonly used)

    (1) Phenothiazine group

        (a) Chlorpromazine (Thorazine)

        (b) Promazine (Sparine)

        (c) Prochlorperazine (Compazine)

        (d) Trifluoperazine (Stelazine)

        (e) Perphenazine (Trilafon)

        (f) Fluphenazine (Prolixin; Permitil)

        (g) Thioridazine (Mellaril)

        (h) Promethazine (Phenergan): This is not used as an antipsychotic agent, however.

    (2) Butyrophenone derivatives

        (a) Haloperidol (Haldol)

    (3) Thioxanthene Derivatives

        (a) Chlorprothixene (Taractan)

        (b) Thiothixene (Navane)

    (4) Rauwolfia group (used with much less frequency currently than they were in the past)

        (a) Reserpine (Serpasil)

        (b) Rescinnamine (Moderil)

        (c) Deserpidine (Harmonyl)

d. List of minor tranquilizers (most commonly used)

    (1) Dial-carbamate group

        (a) Meprobamate (Equanil or Miltown)

        (b) Phenaglycodol (Ultran)

    (2) Diphenylmethane group

        (a) Hydroxyzine (Atarax)

        (b) Hydroxyzine pamoate (Vistaril)

        (c) Benactyzine (Suavitil)

      (3) Benzodiazepine derivatives
         (a) Chlordiazepoxide (Librium)
         (b) Diazepam (Valium)
         (c) Oxazepam (Serax)
         (d) Clorazepate Dipotassium (Tranxene)

D. Antidepressant drugs

1. These drugs are used for treatment of psychiatric depressions. They have been developed intensively during the last few years. Treatment with these drugs is based on the theory that in depressive illness, there is a relative lack, or absence of, catecholamines in the brain, the synthesis of which is affected by antidepressant drugs via different methods.

2. These drugs relieve depression either by direct stimulation, such as produced by the amphetamines, by "bimodal" stimulation, that is, direct and indirect such as produced by the monoamine oxidase inhibitors (MAO), and by indirect stimulation, such as produced by the iminodibenzyl derivatives.

3. Since severe restrictions have been placed on the MAO inhibitors because of the relationship between diet and hypertensive side effects, the iminodibenzyl derivatives have become the principal agents to treat depression.

4. Since the advent of the newer antidepressants, the use of EST for depression has probably decreased.

5. Classification of antidepressive drugs[4]
  a. Hydrazines (MAO inhibitors)
    (1) Isocarboxazid (Marplan)
    (2) Nialamide (Niamid)
    (3) Phenelzine (Nardil)
  b. Nonhydrazine (MAO inhibitor)
    (1) Tranylcypromine (Parnate). From the clinical point of view, this has been by far the most effective antidepressant of this group.
  c. Amphetamines
    (1) Amphetamine (Benzedrine)
    (2) D-Amphetamine (Dexedrine)
  d. Iminodibenzyl derivatives
    (1) Amitriptyline (Elavil)
    (2) Imipramine (Tofranil, Presamine)
    (3) Nortriptyline hydrochloride (Aventyl)

[4]Ibid.

(4) Desipramine hydrochloride (Norpramin, Pertofrane)

(5) Protriptyline (Vivactil)

(6) Doxepin Hydrochloride (Sinequan)

e. Miscellaneous group

(1) Methylphenidate (Ritalin)

(2) Deanol (Deaner)

(3) Benactyzine and meprobamate (in combination marketed as Deprol)

E. Lithium carbonate

1. Lithium has been used widely in some countries for the treatment of psychotic excitements, especially elated episodes.

2. It has been found to be the most effective agent available in treating acute manic episodes. In acute schizophrenic episodes in which a significant affective component is present, it is highly effective in treating the affective component in combination with a phenothiazine.

3. It is also being used to prevent future episodes of elation and depression in people who have manic-depressive illness. Its effectiveness in such a maintenance program is becoming more widely documented.

4. It is also being tried in people who have relapsing depressions. It may be most effective in these depressions when combined with a tricyclic antidepressant such as imipramine.

5. Awareness must be maintained throughout treatment with Lithium salts that thyroid function could possibly be altered and therefore the thyroid function as well as serum lithium levels must be monitored.

F. Use of drugs. Drugs must be integrated into the total treatment program. Drugs by themselves are rarely the entire treatment regime. They often make it possible for a person to participate in his usual activities and also to participate in psychotherapy.

IX. **Management therapy:** There are a number of activities apart from formal psychotherapy and the somatic therapies that have psychotherapeutic value. Among these are the following:

A. Attitude therapy: This is an attempt to prescribe the attitude that all the staff and personnel will assume toward a patient. For example:

1. An attitude of indifference is often therapeutically effective in the management of certain conversion reactions.

2. A firm but nonpunitive attitude is often necessary in managing the antisocial person.
3. A reassuring attitude may be necessary for patients who are anxious and fearful.

B. Occupational therapy: There are many occupational activities which when properly prescribed have psychotherapeutic value. For example:
   1. The use of the punching bag to aid in relieving hostile and aggressive feelings.
   2. Prescribing menial and monotonous tasks to satisfy a need for punishment in a depressed person.
   3. The use of rug weaving, leather working, or painting to satisfy creative and egotistical needs.

C. Recreational therapy: As with occupational therapy, there are a number of recreational activities which also can be of psychotherapeutic value. Recreational activities are of therapeutic value only when they are prescribed to meet certain personality needs and not merely because the person may enjoy them. For example:
   1. Playing baseball may be prescribed for a patient because he needs a means of expressing hostility in a group setting.
   2. Dancing may be prescribed for a shy man to aid him in relating to women.

D. Psychodrama: Here patients dramatize their emotional problems in a group setting. A leading proponent of this therapy is Moreno.

X. Behavior therapy[5]

A. Background
   1. Pavlov, late in his career, attempted to give an account of human psychiatric disorders in terms of excitation and inhibition, the concepts which had so successfully accounted for data from his animal laboratory. His clinical interpretations were less successful but he did stimulate other experimental scientists of learning to apply their analyses to clinical disorders.
   2. Watson (1920) and Jones (1924) demonstrated how a focal fear or phobia could be learned and removed through principles of classical conditioning but these demonstra-

---

[5]Behavior therapy has a specific meaning when used by some writers but will be used here as a general term which refers to all therapies which are derived from theories of learning. (See section on "Behavioral Concepts.") By Shirley H. Mink, Ph.D. and Walter D. Mink, Ph.D.

tions had no significant impact on the practice or theory of clinical psychiatry.

3. Psychologists working with "habit" problems of children (e.g., nail-biting, bed-wetting, temper tantrums, etc.) during the 1920s and 1930s developed practical techniques which are now viewed as forms of behavior therapy.

4. Learning theorists such as O. H. Mowrer (1950), Neal Miller and John Dollard (1950) attempted interpretations of psychoanalytic theory and therapy in terms of the systematic learning theory of Clark Hull (1943) which led to a renewal of the interest of some experimental psychologists of learning the problems of psychiatric disorders.

5. The publication by Joseph Wolpe in 1958 of his book *Psychotherapy by Reciprocal Inhibition*, attracted widespread attention to developments in therapy which had been going on in several countries and signaled the beginning of the modern era of behavior therapy.

6. B. F. Skinner and his student Ogden Lindsley (1954) applied methods of operant learning analysis to the behavior of schizophrenics, and this incursion into the realm of psychiatric disorder was rapidly followed by the application of the same methods to treatment or, in operant conditioning terminology, behavior modification.

B. General principles

1. Behavior therapy can be defined as response modification involving the application of experimentally established principles of learning.

2. Maladaptive behavior is viewed as either deficient or excessive so therapy involves increasing appropriate behaviors that are lacking and decreasing behaviors that are inappropriate in frequency, duration or place of occurrence.

3. Maladaptive responses may be covert as well as overt so such traditional symptoms as hallucinations, delusions, and fantasies are not, in principle, recalcitrant to behavior therapy.

4. Psychiatric disorders are viewed primarily (though not exclusively) as problems of faulty learning.

5. Treatment is directed toward the removal of the inappropriate behaviors, which are viewed traditionally as symptoms, and upon learning new, more effective patterns of behavior.

6. Emphasis in treatment is placed particularly on the current

social environment as a source of stimuli which support symptoms but which can also support changes in behavior.

7. The experimental study of learning and the clinical practice of behavior therapy are viewed as mutually supporting activities which together can contribute to a unified understanding of learned behaviors.

C. Types of behavior therapy: There are many variants of behavior therapy but the three examples that follow typify the most widely used techniques.

1. Systematic desensitization
    a. The technique was developed by Joseph Wolpe (1958) as a means of associating anxiety-eliciting stimuli with responses of relaxation.
    b. Since anxiety and relaxation are incompatible reactions, the increase in the strength of relaxation responses will inhibit the anxiety responses to the same stimuli.
    c. Wolpe's approach consists of three stages:
        (1) Relaxation training similar to the procedures introduced by Jacobson in 1938 in which the subject is taught to identify and control localized tension and relaxation of muscle groups.
        (2) Construction of anxiety hierarchies by the subject in which stimuli or events in the subject's life are ordered from weakest noticeable reactions to them, to strongest.
        (3) Desensitization proper in which the subject in a deep state of relaxation is first presented with an item from the weak end of the hierarchy and then successively stronger ones as the subject is able to maintain anxiety-free relaxation.
    d. Variations of this "gradual-approach" method have also been used to rehearse adequate behaviors in an anxiety-inhibiting context (e.g., sexual arousal, assertiveness).

2. Aversion therapy
    a. This is the oldest of the three procedures that are outlined in this section but it was used for many years with little systematic attention to the conditions of learning which were applied.
    b. The principles of this therapy are straightforward classical (Pavlovian) conditioning procedures in which stimuli associated with a response are conditioned to

some strong unacceptable response such as nausea, pain reactions or extreme disgust.

c. The noxious stimuli which are used to produce the response of aversion may be chemical (e.g., apomorphine), electrical, or visual (including imaginal).

d. The usual application of aversion therapies has been in the therapy of habitual excesses such as overuse of alcohol, and compulsive unacceptable or criminal social behavior such as shoplifting or exhibitionism.

e. Considerable controversy has been generated both about the effectiveness of aversion therapy and the social appropriateness of aversive control of socially deviant behavior. (The novel and movie, *A Clockwork Orange*, provide examples of the social concern about aversive control of behavior.)

f. At present both operant conditioning analyses of the effects of aversive stimuli and the exploration of the effects of aversive imagery represent attempts to find less unpleasant and more socially acceptable alternatives to traditional methods of aversion therapy.

3. Behavior modification (operant methods)

a. Behavior modification represents the application of operant conditioning principles to the interpretation and management of behavioral problems.

b. The basic principle of behavior modification is the control of the reinforcing consequences of behavior; these may range from physical reinforcers such as food to social reinforcers such as approval or tokens of exchange.

c. Behavior modification procedures have been applied in a variety of institutional settings to a great variety of problems.

d. Striking examples of use include language training of autistic children, self-care training of intellectually retarded children and adults, and socialization of regressed psychotic patients.

e. Currently some wards of psychiatric hospitals and some entire institutions are managed according to operant conditioning principles in a *Token-Economy* in which appropriate changes in behavior are rewarded with token reinforcers which can be exchanged for food, activities, and privileges.

f. Behavior modification represents the most active, rapidly expanding and enthusiastically professed of any learning approach to therapy.

4. Evaluation
   a. While behavior therapies were initially developed and applied in the treatment of phobias and compulsions they do not appear to be limited to reactions in which the symptom clearly fits a learning interpretation.
   b. Since the emphasis in treatment is on symptom modification the question of symptom substitution has been raised by some critics (i.e., the removal of one symptom may lead to another if the "cause" is not treated also). However symptom substitution does not occur in most cases according to proponents.
   c. Some enthusiastic supporters of behavior therapy such as Hans Eysenck (1952) claim that their evaluations show behavior therapies to be clearly superior to other forms of psychotherapy particularly psychoanalysis.
   d. More moderate and well-controlled evaluation studies indicate that behavior therapy is a useful treatment procedure and may have particular benefits in situations where environments can be managed to the benefit of patients as in institutions and group living situations.
   e. Since experimental investigations of learning and clinical applications of behavior therapy make use of similar concepts and sources of evidence a consistent association between laboratory and clinic is maintained in this approach to treatment.

REFERENCES

Benson, W. M., and Schiele, B. C. *Tranquilizing and Antidepressive Drugs.* Springfield, Illinois: Charles C. Thomas, Publisher, 1962.

Bergin, A. E., and Garfield, S. L., eds. *Handbook of Psychotherapy and Behavior Change.* New York: John C. Wiley & Sons, Inc., 1971.

Ewalt, Jack R., and Farnsworth, Dana L. *Textbook of Psychiatry.* New York: McGraw-Hill Book Company, 1963.

Franks, C. M. *Behavior Therapy: Appraisal and Status.* New York: McGraw-Hill Book Company, 1969.

Kalinowsky, L. B., and Hoch, P. H. *Somatic Treatment in Psychiatry.* New York: Grune & Stratton, Inc., 1961.

Kolb, L. C. *Modern Clinical Psychiatry.* 8th ed. Philadelphia: W. B. Saunders Company, 1973.

Lunzer, Richard G. Personal communication on group therapy, February 1969.

Schiele, B. C., and Benson, W. M. "Tranquilizing and Related Drugs: A Guide for the General Physician." *Postgraduate Medicine* 23(May 1958): 484.

Yates, A. J. *Behavior Therapy.* New York: John C. Wiley & Sons, Inc., 1970.

Glossary

Abstinence Syndrome—The withdrawal symptoms which develop when addicting drugs are withheld.

Acrophobia—Fear of heights.

Addiction—Involves three phenomena: tolerance, habituation, and physical dependence.

Affect—Mood or feeling tone.

Affective Disorder—A personality disorder in which the fundamental disturbance is in the mood (affect).

Agitation—A state of restlessness and uneasiness; mental perturbation; typically found in involutional melancholia.

Agoraphobia—Fear of open spaces.

Alcoholism—A personality disorder characterized by excessive use of alcohol to the point of habituation, overdependence, or addiction.

Alcoholics Anonymous (AA)—This is an informal worldwide fellowship of groups of alcoholics who help each other to stay sober and to remain abstinent.

Alzheimer's Disease—A degenerative organic brain disease generally occurring in middle life.

Ambivalence—The coexistence of two opposing feelings toward the same individual or object; they may be conscious, unconscious, or partly both.

Amnesia—Pathological memory loss.

Amok—An acute outburst of violence or murderous frenzy, usually found in Malayan men.

Anancastic Personality (anal personality)—*See* Obsessive Compulsive Personality.

Anaclitic—Dependency on others; as for example, the dependent relationship the infant has with his mother.

Anal Stage—From the eighteenth month until the end of the third year; the infant's attention is centered on bowel and excretory functions.

Anima—The true inner-self or soul.

Anorexia Nervosa—A syndrome found in young people, characterized by marked, prolonged appetite loss with accompanying marked weight loss (psychogenic malnutrition).

Antecendent Factors—Forces operating during the early developmental years.

Antidepressant—A drug used in the treatment of psychiatric depressions.

Antisocial Personality—A person who is basically unsocialized and whose behavior patterns bring him into repeated conflict with society. Sociopathic personality. Psychopathic Personality.

Anxiety—Uneasiness, apprehension, or fearfulness stemming from anticipated danger, the source of which is unidentifiable.

Anxiety Neurosis—A reaction in which anxiety is the most prominent feature.

Apathy—Lack of feeling, emotion, interest, or concern.

Asthenic Personality—A personality type characterized by easy fatigability, lasitude, low energy level, lack of enthusiam, marked incapacity for enjoyment (anhedonia), lack of will (abulia), and oversensitivity to physical and emotional stress.

Autism—Persistent overindulgence in fantasy which ignores reality.

Automatism—Unconscious automatic and apparently unguided symbolic behavior as, for example, automatic handwriting.

Behavior Disorders of Childhood (adolescence)—This category is reserved for disorders occurring in childhood and adolescence that are more stable, internalized, and resistant to treatment than transient situational disturbances, but less so than psychoses, neuroses, and personality disorders.

Behaviorism—John B. Watson's Theory of Psychology which is based on observable behavior rather than unobservable mentalistic functions.

Behavior Therapy—Refers to all therapies which are derived from theories of learning.

Bestiality—Sexual gratification through intercourse with living animals.

Blocking—Difficulty in recalling, or interruption of a stream of speech or thought due to emotional forces which are usually conscious.

Castration Anxiety—Feared loss of male genitals, includes the childhood fantasy that female genitals result from the loss of the penis.

Catalepsy—A generalized diminished responsiveness or immobility characterized by trancelike states.

Catatonic Excitement—A form of schizophrenia characterized by extreme psychomotor agitation; including violent excitement, destructiveness, and assaultiveness; and a continuous incoherent stream of speech.

Catatonic Stupor—A form of schizophrenia characterized by mutism, negativism, stereotypies, echopraxia, mannerisms, posturizing, waxy flexibility, automatic obedience, retention of excretions, and refusal to eat.

Cathexis—The process by which unconscious primitive drives are vested with psychic energy.

Circumstantiality—A state of being incidental, adventitious, and irrelevant in details.

Clarification—A process by which the physician helps the patient better understand his feelings and behavior and to have a clearer picture of external realities.

Claustrophobia—Fear of closed spaces.

Clouding of Consciousness—A condition in which there is impairment of retention, perception, and orientation.

Collective Unconscious—The racial unconscious as distinguished from the *personal* unconscious (Jungian Theory).

Coma (stupor)—A state of unawareness and nonreactiveness.

Compartmentalization—*See* Dissociation.

Compensation—A conscious or unconscious attempt to overcome real or fancied inferiorities.

Compensation Neurosis—A neurotic reaction in which secondary gain factors are conspicuous; the secondary gain may be any external benefit which is derived from the illness; that is, disability benefits, financial gain, or personal attention.

Compulsion—A recurrent compelling act which develops as an attempt to relieve obsessions or fears.

Conation—Basic strivings of an individual as expressed in his actions and behavior.

Concurrent Factors—Precipitating or immediate causes which may trigger or initiate the onset of an acute mental reaction.

Confabulation—A falsification of memory in which actual memory gaps are "filled in" by imaginary experiences (fabricated) which seem plausible and are recounted in detail.

Confusion—Disorientation in respect to time, place, or person; accompanied by a state of perplexity; it is sometimes accompanied by disturbances of consciousness.

Consciousness—Synonymous with awareness.

Conversion Hysteria—*See* Hysterical Neurosis, Conversion Type.

Coprolalia—The compulsive utterance of obscene words.

Coprophagia—A desire to eat feces.

Coprophilia—Sexual interest in excretions.

Countercathexis—The opposition of ego energy to id energy.

Countertransference—The therapist's unconscious or conscious emotional reaction to the patient.

Cryptomnesia—The appearance in consciousness of memory images which are not recognized as such but which appear as original experiences or creations.

Cunnilingus—Sexual activity in which the mouth and tongue are employed to stimulate the female genitals.

Cyclothymic Personality—A personality type characterized by recurring and alternating periods of depression and elation. Sometimes described as miniature manic-depressive illness.

Defense Mechanisms—Specific, unconscious, intrapsychic adjustive efforts which are utilized to resolve emotional conflict and free the individual from anxiety.

Déjà vu—A subjective sensation that an experience which is really happening for the first time occurred on a previous occasion.

Delirium—A condition characterized by disorientation in all three spheres, obvious mood changes such as anxiousness, fearfulness or excitement, illusions, and vivid hallucinations.

Delirium Tremens (DT'S)—An acute psychotic episode characterized by delirium, coarse tremors, and frightening visual hallucinations usually becoming more intense in the dark.

Delusion—A fixed false belief that is not in keeping with the individual's cultural or educational level.

Dementia—Organic loss of intellectual function.

Denial—The unconscious disavowal of thoughts, feelings, wishes, needs, or external reality factors which are consciously unacceptable.

Depersonalization—Feelings of unreality, strangeness, or altered identity.

Depersonalization Neurosis—A disorder of affect in which the person has feelings of unreality, altered personality, or altered identity.

Depression—A feeling of sadness, loneliness, dejection, or hopelessness.

Depressive Neurosis—A pathological state of sadness in which the etiological factor is less obvious than in normal grief, or the depression is more severe, or persists unduly long.

Deterioration—Progressive loss of intellectual and emotional functions.

Disorientation—Loss of awareness of one's position in relationship to time, one's surroundings, or relationships with other persons.

Displacement—The redirection of an emotion from the original object to a more acceptable substitute object.

Dissociation—The unconscious detachment of certain behavior or personality activities from the normal or usual conscious behavior patterns of an individual, which then function alone (compartmentalization).

Dissociative Reaction—*See* Hysterical Neurosis, Dissociative Type.

Dream State—A transient clouding of consciousness of intrapsychic origin in which the person is unaware of his surroundings and behaves violently or opposite to his usual pattern.

Drug Dependence—Marked emotional or physiological dependence on drugs to a point beyond voluntary control.

Dual Personality—*See* Multiple Personality.

Dyssocial Behavior—An individual in this group shows disregard for the usual social and moral codes and often comes in conflict with them as the result of having lived all or most of his life in an abnormal moral environment.

Echolalia—The pathological repetition of phrases or words of another person.

Echopraxia—The repetition or imitation of movements the subject is observing.

Ecstasy—A feeling of intense rapture found in states of depersonalization and psychoses such as schizophrenia.

Ego—The part of the personality which meets and interacts with the outside world.

Eidetic Imagery—The ability to produce vivid, accurate, and detailed visual after-images; "photographic memory."

Elation—Marked euphoria accompanied by increased motor activity.

Electroshock (electroconvulsive) Therapy—A form of psychiatric treatment in which sufficient electrical current is passed through electrodes applied to both temporal areas of the head to produce a grand mal seizure.

Environmental Modification (environmental manipulation)—Changing the environment in any way.

Eros—The creative forces; the life instinct.

Euphoria—An exaggerated sense of well-being not consistent with the reality situation.

Exhibitionism—Exposure of one's body, especially the genitalia as a means of attracting sexual attention or achieving sexual excitement or gratification.

Explosive Personality—A personality type characterized by uncontrollable gross outbursts of rage or of verbal or physical aggressiveness.

Extrapsychic—From the environment or, external world forces.

Extroversion—Outwardly directed libido (away from one's self).

Exultation—Intense elation accompanied by grandiosity.

Family Therapy—Psychotherapy in which the focus is on the family with one or more therapists dealing with an entire family unit. The goal is to resolve or reduce the pathogenic conflicts and anxiety within the unit.

Fantasy—Fabricated series of mental pictures or sequence of events; daydreaming.

Fellatio—Oral stimulation of the penis.

Fetishism—Sexual excitement or gratification derived from substitution of some inanimate object, or some part of the body for a human love object.

Fixation—The arrest of maturation at an earlier level of psychosexual development.

Flight of Ideas—Skipping from one idea to another in quick succession, but without reaching the goal idea.

Folle À Deux—A psychotic disorder in which two closely related people, usually members of the same family and who live in close intimate association, mutually share identical delusions.

Frottage—Sexual pleasure from rubbing or pressing against fully clothed members of the opposite sex.

Fugue State—A personality dissociation characterized by memory loss and flight from the immediate environment.

Functional Psychoses—Psychotic reactions which are not caused by any known physical condition.

Ganser Syndrome—An emotional reaction, occurring chiefly in prisoners, which is characterized by childish, ludicrous behavior; nonsense syndrome; prison psychosis; syndrome of approximate answers.

Genital Stage—The final phase of psychosexual development.

Grief (bereavement)—A normal, appropriate, affective sadness in response to a recognizable external loss.

Group Psychotherapy (several individuals take part)—Use of psychotherapeutic techniques in group setting, and the utilization of group interaction.

Hallucination—Sensory perceptions which have no actual stimuli.

Hebephrenic Schizophrenia—A form of schizophrenia characterized by marked regression to primitive, unorganized, and uninhibited behavior.

Holism—*See* Psychobiology.

Homosexuality—Sexual attraction or desire for sexual contact with a person of the same sex.

Hostility—anger, antagonism, opposition, or resistance in thought or behavior.

Huntington's Chorea—A degenerative disease of the basal ganglia and cerebral cortex.

Hypermnesia—Abnormally vivid or complete memory, or the reawakening of impressions long seemingly forgotten.

Hyperventilation Syndrome—A condition in which the individual is subject to repeated forced respirations, yawning, sensations of air hunger, occasional tetany, chest pain, light-headedness, parasthesias of the hands, feet, and face, and an intense conviction of impending death.

Hypnagogic Hallucinations—Mental images that sometimes occur just before sleep.

Hypnopompic Hallucinations—Images seen in dreams which persist on awakening.

Hypnotherapy—The use of hypnosis as a means of facilitating psychotherapy.

Hypochondrical Neurosis (hypochondriasis)—A neurosis characterized by persistent and obsessive preoccupation with physical or emotional health, and accompanied by various somatic symptoms without demonstrated organic cause.

Hysterical Neurosis, Conversion Type—A neurotic disorder in which unconscious conflict is manifested as disguised and symbolic somatic symptoms. The anxiety arising out of some conflictual situation is converted into somatic symptoms in parts of the body innervated by the sensorimotor system. (Symbolic Somatization.)

Hysterical Neurosis, Dissociative Type—A neurotic reaction in which there is an automatic unconscious separation, splitting-off, or detachment of certain functions or parts of the personality.

Hysterical Personality (histrionic personality disorder)—A personality disorder characterized by excitability, emotional instability, overreactivity, and self-dramatization.

Id—The unconscious part of the personality which serves as the reservoir of primitive drives (instincts).

Idealization—The over-estimation of admired qualities of another person or desired object.

Identification—The unconscious, wishful adoption (internalization) of the personality characteristics or identity of another individual, generally one possessing attributes which the subject envies or admires.

Illusions—Misinterpretation of real external sensory experiences (usually optical or auditory).

Impulse Neurosis (impulse-ridden state)—A neurotic character or acting out neurotic whose disturbance is characterized by the irresistible, repetitious expression of a single, pleasurable impulse.

Inadequate Personality—A personality type characterized by ineffectual responses to emotional, social, intellectual, and physical demands.

Inappropriativeness—Affect opposite to what would be expected. Observed in schizophrenia.

Incest—Sexual relations between members of the same family.

Incoherence—Disorderly, illogical thought progression.

Incorporation—A primitive defense mechanism in which the psychic image of a person is wholly or partially assimilated into an individual's personality.

Inferiority Complex—The conflict, partly conscious and partly unconscious, which impels the individual to make attempts to overcome the distress accompanying inferiority feelings.

Insight—The degree to which the patient can appreciate the nature of his condition and need for treatment.

Insulin Coma Therapy—A form of psychiatric treatment in which regular insulin is injected daily in increasing doses until hypoglycemic coma results.

Intellectualization—The overuse of intellectual concepts and words to avoid affective experience or expression of feeling.

Intelligence Quotient (IQ)—A common measure of intelligence arrived at by dividing the mental age achieved on a test by chronological age and multiplying the result by 100.

Intelligence Test—Standardized means of assessing a person's current mental abilities, e.g., the Stanford-Binet Test and the Wechsler Adult Intelligence Scale.

Intrapsychic—From within the personality.

Introversion—Inwardly directed libido, reflected in the tendency to be preoccupied with one's self.

Involutional Melancholia—A psychotic reaction with initial onset in the involutional period (late middle life).

Involutional Paranoid State (involutional paraphrenia)—A paranoid psychosis with initial onset of delusion formation in the involutional period.

Isolation—The separation of an unacceptable impulse, act, or idea from its memory origin, thereby removing the emotional charge associated with the original memory.

Kleptomania—Neurotic stealing.

Korsakov's Psychosis—A chronic brain syndrome characterized by amnesia, disorientation, confabulation, and peripheral neuropathy.

Latency Period—Middle childhood, the stage between the oedipal period and adolescence.

Latent Homosexuality—Homosexual desires are largely unconscious, unrecognized, and sublimated.

Lesbianism—Homosexual behavior in females.

Libido—The emotional energy broadly derived from the underlying instincts (psychosexual energy) and presumably present at birth.

Lithium—A salt used in the treatment of psychotic excitements, especially elated episodes.

Lobotomy (frontal lobotomy)—This is the most commonly used of the psychosurgical procedures and consists of sectioning the frontal lobes of the brain.

Logorrhea—Uncontrollable, rapid, excessive talking.

Magical Thinking—Belief that thinking becomes reality ("wishing will make it so").

Malingering—Conscious simulation of illness utilized as an avoidance of an unpleasant or intolerable alternative.

Management Therapy—Those activities apart from formal psychotherapy and the somatic therapies that have psychotherapeutic value.

Manic-Depressive Illness—A psychotic reaction characterized by severe mood swings—elation and depression—and a tendency to remission and recurrence.

Mannerisms—Stereotyped movements such as blinking, grimacing, gesturing, etc.

Masochism—Sexual pleasure from enduring physical or psychological pain (may be inflicted by one's self or by others).

Masculine Protest—Male and female attempts to escape from the feminine, submissive role.

Migraine—A syndrome characterized by recurrent, severe unilateral cephalgia (headache), nausea, vomiting, and scotomata (visual disturbances).

Minnesota Multiphasic Personality Inventory (MMPI)—The most widely used objective personality test which consists of an inventory of 550 true-false items.

Misidentification—Incorrect identification of other people.

Mutilple Personality—The unconscious adoption of two or more different personalities which are separate and compartmentalized. Generally, the primary character is proper and moral while the secondary personality is hedonistic and impulse-ridden.

Mutism—A form of negativism characterized by refusal to speak for conscious or unconscious reasons.

Narcoanalysis (narcosynthesis)—Interviewing a patient under intravenously administered barbiturates.

Necrophilia—Sexual gratification from corpses.

Negativism—Opposition, resistance, or refusal to accept reasonable suggestions or advice and a tendency to be oppositional.

Neologism—A coined word or condensation of several words to express a complex idea which has a special meaning to that person.

Neurasthenic Neurosis (neurasthenia)—A neurosis characterized by symptoms of weakness, marked fatigability, overwhelming exhaustion, poor concentration, feelings of inadequacy, and an exaggerated attention to bodily organs and functions.

Neurosis—Maladaptive emotional state resulting from unresolved, unconscious conflicts.

Obsession—A persistent, recurring idea or impulse that remains in consciousness despite its irrationality.

Obsessive-Compulsive Neurosis—A neurosis characterized by obsessions (persistent, recurring ideas or impulses that remain in consciousness despite their irrationality) and compulsions (illogical, repetitive, and undesired urges to perform acts which are against the person's ordinary wishes).

Obsessive-Compulsive Personality—A personality type characterized by excessive concern with conformity and adherence to standards of conscience.

Oedipus Complex—In Freudian Theory the attachment of the young child for the parent of the opposite sex, accompanied by envious and aggressive feelings toward the parent of the same sex.

Oral Stage—The first twelve to eighteen months of life which are characterized chiefly by preoccupation with the feeding experience.

Organic Brain Syndromes—Mental disorder caused by or associated with impairment of brain tissue function.

Orientation—Awareness of one's relationship to time, place, and identity of person.

Overt Homosexuality—Homosexuality which is recognized consciously.

Panic—An acute anxiety attack of overwhelming severity which leads to disorganization of ego functions.

Paramnesia—Distortion or falsification of memory in which the individual confuses reality and fantasy.

Paranoia—A psychotic disorder characterized by an elaborate, well-systematized, complex, intricate, logical, and well-fixed delusional system but with relatively good preservation of the remainder of the personality.

Paranoid Personality—A personality type characterized by hypersensitivity, rigidity, unwarranted suspicion, jealousy, envy, excessive self-importance, and a tendency to blame others and ascribe evil motives to them.

Paranoid Schizophrenia—A form of schizophrenia characterized by paranoid delusions that are "illogical" and unsystematized, usually of a persecutory nature, but may be grandiose.

Paranoid States—Psychotic disorders in which a delusion, generally persecutory or grandiose, is the essential abnormality (DSM-II). They are usually without hallucinations or schizophrenic behavior.

Paraphrenia—A disorder characterized by paranoid delusions without deterioration, dementia or loss of contact with reality, other than in the area of the delusional system.

Passive-Aggressive Personality—A personality type characterized by both passivity and aggressivity. The aggressiveness may be expressed in such passive ways as obstructionism, pouting, procrastination, intentional inefficiency, or stubbornness.

Pederasty—Anal intercourse between a man and a boy.

Pedophilia—Pathological sexual interest in children of the same or opposite sex.

Perception—The awareness and intended integration of sensory impressions of the environment and the interpretation of them in the light of experience.

Perseveration—A persistent, repetitive expression of a single idea in response to various questions.

Persona—The social facade assumed by an individual (so named from the mask worn by actors in ancient Greek drama which characterized the mood portrayed).

Personality—The sum total of the individual's internal and external patterns of adjustment to life.

Personality Disorders—Disorders characterized by deeply ingrained, maladaptive behavioral patterns that are lifelong in duration and often recognizable at adolescence or earlier.

Phallic Stage—This period extends from the end of the third year to the seventh year; the child becomes aware of his or her genitalia.

Pharmacotherapy—The treatment of psychiatric conditions with drugs.

Phobia—Persistent, obsessive fear of a specific object or situation.

Phobic Neurosis—A reaction characterized by a persistent, obsessive fear of a specific object or situation.

Pick's Disease—A presenile degenerative disease of the brain affecting the cerebral cortex, particularly the frontal lobes.

Pleasure Principle—The seeking of pleasure and the avoidance of pain.

Porphyria—An episodic metabolic disorder characterized by the excretion of porphyrine in the urine and accompanied by attacks of abdominal pain, peripheral neuropathy, and acute psychotic manifestations.

Posturizing—The assumption of an unusual posture which is maintained over a prolonged period of time.

Pregenital Stage—The oral and anal stages considered together.

Preoccupation—Extreme or excessive concern with one's thoughts, engrossment.

Primary Gain—Relief of anxiety through the development of neuroses.

Primary Processes—The psychological expressions of the underlying basic drives; assumed to be largely unconscious; present at birth; could be considered innate.

Projection—The attributing to another person or object, thoughts, feelings, motives, or desires which are really one's own disavowed and unacceptable traits.

Psychoanalytic Therapy—The exploration of the unconscious, chiefly through free association.

Psychobiology—Adolf Meyer's psychiatric theory which "studies not only the person as a whole, as a unit, but also the whole man."

Psychobiological Therapy—Critical examination and evaluation of conscious forces in the patient's personality development and emotional problems.

Psychodrama—Patients dramatize their emotional problems in a group setting.

Psychodynamics—The explanation or interpretation of human behavior and mental states in terms of mental or emotional forces.

Psychogenesis—Development from psychological origins as distinguished from physical origins.

Psychogenic—Psychological origin as distinguished from physical cause.

Psychomotor Excitement—Mental and physical hyperactivity.

Psychomotor Retardation—Slowing down of mental and physical activity.

Psychopathology—The study of causes and manifestations of mental disorder.

Psychophysiologic Disorders—A group of reactions characterized by somatic symptoms that result from emotional factors and involve organ systems usually innervated by the autonomic nervous system (which is not under voluntary control).

Psychoses—Major mental disorders in which there is a departure from normal patterns of thinking, feeling and acting; commonly characterized by loss of contact with reality, perceptual distortion, regressive behavior, and attitudes; diminished controls of elementary impulses and desires, abnormal mental content including delusions and hallucinations; may be of organic or emotional origin.

Psychosurgery—A group of surgical procedures directed at certain areas of the brain in an effort to relieve various symptoms of mental illness.

Psychotherapy—This includes everything done to or for a patient that has a favorable effect upon him. Is the generic term for any type of treatment which is based primarily upon verbal or nonverbal communication with the patient as distinguished from the use of drugs, surgery, or physical measure such as electroconvulsive treatment.

Psychotic-Depressive Reaction—This term is reserved for those cases with a depressive mood attributable to some experience in which there is ordinarily no history of repeated depression or cyclothymic mood swings.

Pyromania—Erotic excitement and gratification from starting and watching fires.

Rapport—In psychiatry, the constant feeling of harmonious accord, mutual responsiveness, and sympathy that contributes to the patient's confidence in the therapist and willingness to work cooperatively with him.

Rationalization—The ascribing of acceptable or worthwhile motives to thoughts, feelings, or behavior which really have other unrecognized motives.

Reaction Formation—The direction of overt behavior or attitudes in precisely the opposite direction of the individual's underlying, unacceptable impulses (the underlying impulses may be conscious or unconscious).

Reality Principle—The demands of the external world.

Reassurance—The imparting or restoration of confidence and freeing the patient from fear and anxiety.

Regression—The return to an earlier level of emotional adjustment at which gratification was assured.

Repression—The involuntary, automatic banishment of unacceptable ideas or impulses into the unconscious (motivated unconscious forgetting).

Restitution—A supplantation of a highly valued object that has been lost through rejection by or death or departure of another object.

Retrospective Falsification—Unconscious distortion of past experiences to conform to present emotional needs.

Rorshach Test—A projective test in which the examinee is instructed to interpret a series of ten ink-blots reproduced on cards.

Sadism—Sexual excitement or gratification from inflicting physical pain on others.

Sado-masochism—The occurrence of sadism and masochism in the same person. Sadism and masochism often occur together and Freud regarded masochism as sadism turned inward.

Schizophrenia—A group of disorders manifested by characteristic disturbances of thinking, mood, and behavior. Disturbances in thinking are marked by alterations of concept formation which may lead to misinterpretation of reality and sometimes to deluxions and hallucinations which frequently appear psychologically self-protective. Corollary mood changes include ambivalent, constricted, and inappropriate emotional responsiveness and loss of empathy with others. Behavior may be withdrawn, regressive, and bizarre (DSM-II, 1968).

Schizoid Personality—A personality type characterized by shyness, oversensitivity, seclusiveness, avoidance of close or competitive relationships, and often eccentricity.

Secondary Gain—Is the advantage that accrues to the patient by virtue of his illness; it is most prominent in the hysterical reactions.

Secondary Processes—This refers to the manner in which the underlying basic drives are controlled and permitted expression in reasonable and acceptable ways.

Senium—Period of old age.

Sexual Deviation—Any aberrant sexual behavior which is predominantly preferred to, or takes the place of, normal heterosexual behavior.

Sexual Orientation Disturbance—Individuals whose sexual interests are directed primarily toward people of the same sex and who are either disturbed by, in conflict with, or wish to change their sexual orientation.

Simple Schizophrenia—A form of schizophrenia whose chief characteristics are emotional blunting, apathy, and preoccupation with fantasy life. Sometimes appears intellectually dull. There are no delusions or hallucinations.

Somatization Reaction—Neurotic disorders manifested primarily as physical symptoms.

Somatogenesis—Development from physical (somatic) origins as distinguished from psychological origins.

Somatogenic—Physical or organic cause, as distinguished from psychological origin.

Somnabulism—Sleep walking.

Stereotypy—The persistent repetition of a motor activity.

Stupor—*See* Coma.

Sublimation—The diversion of unacceptable, instinctual drives into socially sanctioned channels.

Substitution—Unconscious replacement of a highly valued but unattainable or unacceptable emotional goal or object by one which is attainable or acceptable.

Superego—The censoring force of the personality.

Supportive Psychotherapy—Deals predominately with conscious material and is centered chiefly on support of the individual strength and assets.

Suppression—The voluntary, intentional relegation of unacceptable ideas or impulses to the foreconscious (preconscious); this is conscious forgetting.

Symbolization—The unconscious mechanism by which a neutral idea or object is used to represent another idea or object which has a forbidden aspect to it.

Thanatos—The aggressive, destructive, or death forces.

Thematic Apperception Test (TAT)—A projective test consisting of a set of twenty black-and-white pictures reproduced on cards, each depicting a potentially emotion-laden situation. The examinee, presented with the cards one at a time, is instructed to make up a story about each situation.

Thinking—Exercising the powers of judgement, conception, or inference as distinguished from sensory perception.

Tranquilizers—Drugs which produce emotional calmness and relaxation without sedation, hypnosis, motor impairment or euphoria. They act principally on the lower brain centers.

Transference—The unconscious attachment to the therapist (or others who have a treatment relationship with the patient) of feelings and attitudes that were originally related to important figures (parents, siblings, etc.) in one's early life.

Transient Situational Disturbances—Disorders which are more or less transient in character and appear to represent an acute reaction to an overwhelming environmental stress in an individual without evident underlying mental disorder.

Transsexualism—A deviancy in which the person is physically normal but has a total aversion to his or her biological sex that dates from early childhood.

Transvestism—Sexual excitation or gratification from wearing the clothing, and enacting the role of the opposite sex.

Uncovering Psychotherapy (intensive psychotherapy, insight therapy)—The aim is to produce insight through uncovering conflicts, chiefly unconscious, and learning to deal with them more effectively.

Undoing—A primitive defense mechanism in which some unacceptable past behavior is symbolically acted out in reverse, usually repetitiously (symbolic atonement).

Ventilation (unburdening)—The therapeutic release of feelings through conscious, free expression.

Verbigeration—Meaningless repetition of incoherent words or sentences.

Voyeurism (scopophilia)—Erotic pleasure from watching others in the nude, usually paying particular attention to the genitalia ("Peeping Tom").

Word-Salad—A mixture of words and pharases which are incomprehensible and incoherent.

Index